Draw Your Feelings

Draw Your Feelings

a creative journal to help connect with your emotions through art

RUKMINI PODDAR

1

Vermilion/Happy Place Books, an imprint of Ebury Publishing
20 Vauxhall Bridge Road
London SW1V 2SA

Vermilion is part of the Penguin Random House group of companies whose addresses
can be found at global.penguinrandomhouse.com

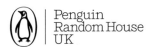

Copyright © Rukmini Poddar 2023

Rukmini Poddar has asserted her right to be identified as the author of this Work in
accordance with the Copyright, Designs and Patents Act 1988

First published by Vermilion/Happy Place Books in 2023

First published in the United States of America in 2023 by TarcherPerigee, an imprint of
Penguin Random House LLC, New York

www.penguin.co.uk

A CIP catalogue record for this book is available from the British Library

ISBN: 9781785044779

Printed and bound in China by C&C Offset Printing Co., Ltd

The authorised representative in the EEA is Penguin Random House Ireland, Morrison
Chambers, 32 Nassau Street, Dublin D02 YH68.

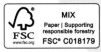

Penguin Random House is committed to a sustainable future for our business, our readers
and our planet. This book is made from Forest Stewardship Council® certified paper.

To all my teachers—
for nurturing my seed of Bhakti
and teaching me to express my heart through art

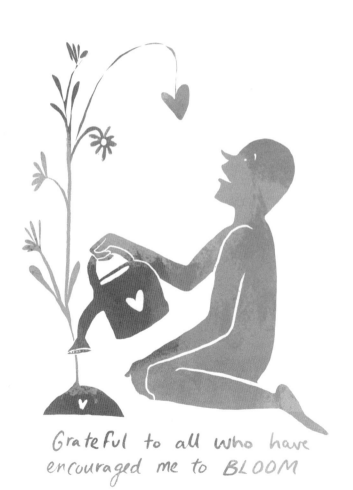

Grateful to all who have
encouraged me to BLOOM

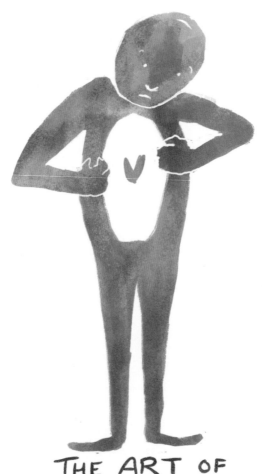

THE ART OF
Trying to
OPEN UP

THIS BOOK BELONGS TO:

Write out your name below. Try it again with your nondominant hand.
Now try writing it with your eyes closed. Or add your thumbprint. The options are endless!

CONTENTS

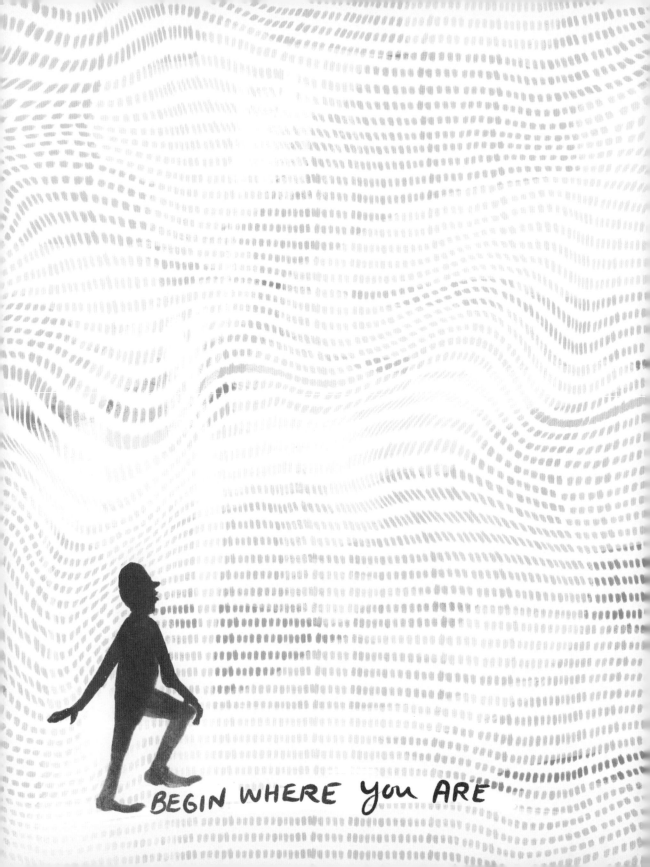

BEGIN WHERE you ARE

INTRODUCTION

preparing for
your creative journey ahead

the most important **journey**
you will ever take
is the one **inside** of you

WHY DRAW YOUR FEELINGS?

I like to say that I accidentally stumbled into my illustration career in 2016 when I decided to draw my own obscure emotions and share them online. What started off as a personal project ended up taking on a life of its own.

Drawing my feelings allowed me to get back in touch with my voice. To create meaning out of emotions that otherwise felt confusing and indescribable.

When I shared what was deeply personal for me, I was able to tune in to what was universally felt by others. I soon realized that we are not alone in how we feel.

I believe creativity is a way for us to come back to ourselves. When we are lost, we use our voice to call for help. The same goes for your creative voice: When you learn to use it to express how you feel, you can transform the way you relate with yourself, others, and the world around you.

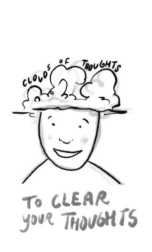

TO CLEAR YOUR THOUGHTS

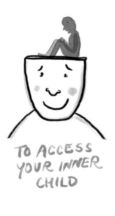

TO ACCESS YOUR INNER CHILD

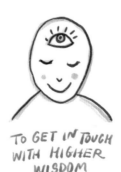

TO GET IN TOUCH WITH HIGHER WISDOM

TO FIND BEAUTY IN THE MUNDANE

change your relationship
TO YOUR EMOTIONS

Emotions are that invisible source of energy that guides your life.

You wear your feelings like you wear a pair of tinted lenses—they color and filter how you see the world. Emotions can empower, but they can also control. Change your relationship to your emotions and you'll change how you experience the world.

This book will help you journey deep within yourself—first to connect with your emotions, and then to change the way you live with them.

The journey helps us to shed the layers of our false identity and limited beliefs. We can finally accept parts of ourselves that have long been neglected. We have stepped away from our own stories—if only for a moment—to see a larger perspective.

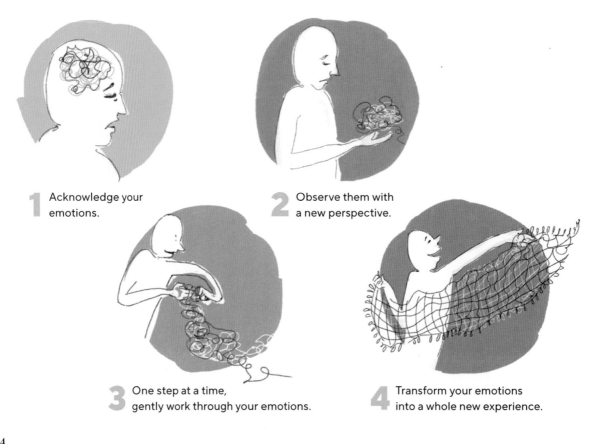

1 Acknowledge your emotions.

2 Observe them with a new perspective.

3 One step at a time, gently work through your emotions.

4 Transform your emotions into a whole new experience.

Pause and EXPERIENCE your EMOTIONS from A NEW PERSPECTIVE

Healthy distance leads to healthy perspective. Your emotions are a huge part of your experience, but they are not *who* you are. This distinction is important. What was once overwhelming can seem small with the right perspective. Healthy detachment starts with realizing *who you are not,* adjusting your perspective, and becoming an *active observer of your life.*

WAYS I HANDLE MY EMOTIONS

COMPARTMENTALIZE

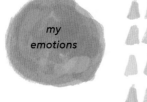
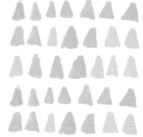

my emotions

the rest of my life

SUPPRESS

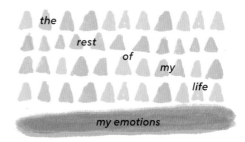

the rest of my life

my emotions

SPILL OVER

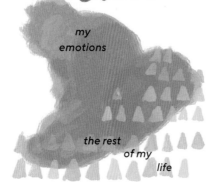

my emotions

the rest of my life

OVERWHELM

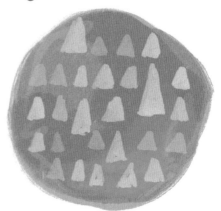

my emotions = my life

How do you usually regulate your emotions? There are two extremes when it comes to managing your emotions: Either you suppress your feelings and compartmentalize them . . . or you lose all control and allow your emotions to overwhelm you fully. But there is a middle way—integrating your emotions through healthy self-expression.

HOW MUCH CAN THE HEART EXPAND?

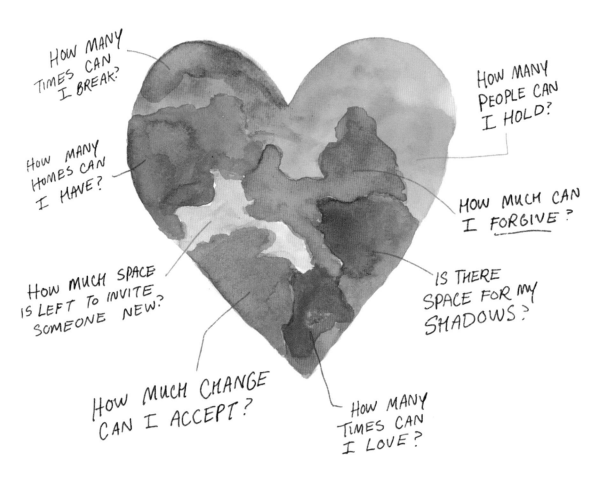

HOW MANY TIMES CAN I BREAK?

HOW MANY HOMES CAN I HAVE?

HOW MUCH SPACE IS LEFT TO INVITE SOMEONE NEW?

HOW MUCH CHANGE CAN I ACCEPT?

HOW MANY PEOPLE CAN I HOLD?

HOW MUCH CAN I FORGIVE?

IS THERE SPACE FOR MY SHADOWS?

HOW MANY TIMES CAN I LOVE?

Integrating your emotions means allowing your heart to hold *all* your feelings. The good news is that your heart has the capacity to hold it all. Your heart has broken and repaired itself countlessly. Only through acknowledging and accepting your emotions can you access and continuously expand your heart's capacity to feel.

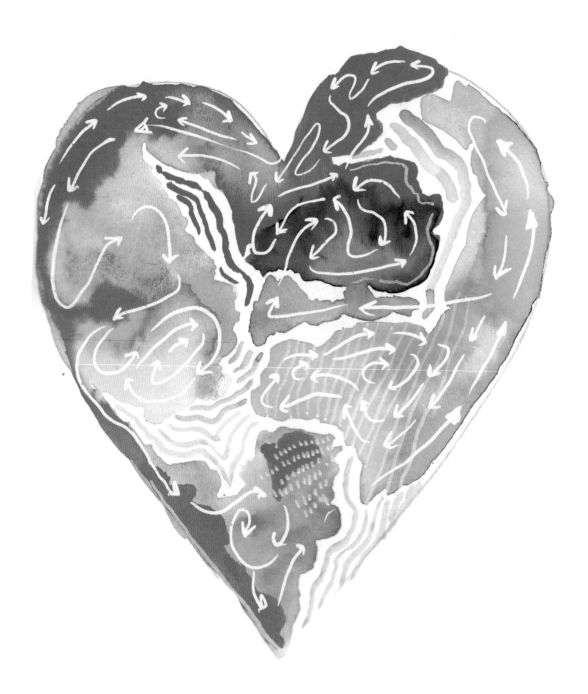

Imagine that each chapter of this book is a different area of your heart. As you journey through each chapter, you will build skills and learn more about yourself. Each chapter builds on the previous one. The chapter guide on the next page gives you a glance of what's to come.

Chapter Guide

 Chapter 1: Emotions as Visual Art
Get started with the basics: line, pattern, shape, color, and scale

 Chapter 2: Emotions as Form
Learn the simplest way to draw emotions expressed through the body

 Chapter 3: Emotions as Metaphor
Use symbols and metaphors to draw what is otherwise invisible to the eye

 Chapter 4: Emotions as Data
Learn how to find emotional meaning within data—and turn it into art

 Chapter 5: PAUSE
Slow down and congratulate yourself—you have officially made it halfway!

 Chapter 6: Your Relationship to Your Parts
Go deeper into your relationship with yourself by understanding your parts

 Chapter 7: Your Relationship to Others
Reflect and visualize the many ways you relate with other people in your life

 Chapter 8: Your Relationship to Your Values
Recognize and draw out your core values—and how they show up in your life

 Chapter 9: Accepting All Your Emotions
Learn the wisdom of what ALL your emotions are teaching you

 Chapter 10: EXHALE
Celebrate all the ways you have grown with a deep, long exhale

creativity is your **birthright**

Claim your creative voice and express your emotions.

WAYS TO WELCOME THE NEW

How can you prepare for your creative journey? The most important preparation is to shift your mindset from being an achiever to being a receiver. The goal of this workbook is to practice openness, acceptance, and patience. Starting where you are is the most important prerequisite you need.

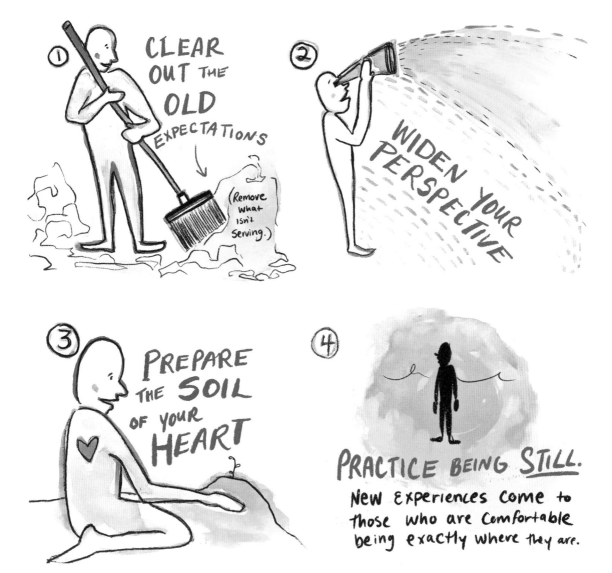

① CLEAR OUT THE OLD EXPECTATIONS
(Remove what isn't serving.)

② WIDEN YOUR PERSPECTIVE

③ PREPARE THE SOIL OF YOUR HEART

④ PRACTICE BEING STILL.
New experiences come to those who are comfortable being exactly where they are.

CHALLENGES TO EXPECT

No journey is without its challenges. By acknowledging what will get in the way, we can create strategies to work through them. Can you recognize and name what your own challenges will be?

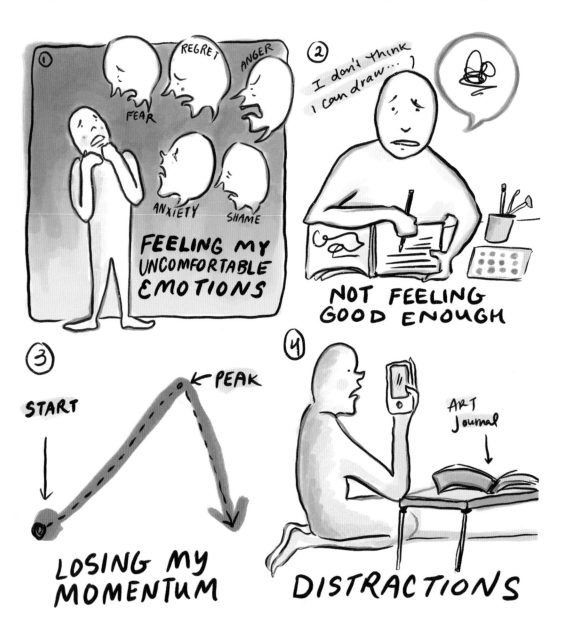

BENEFITS to EXPECT

We stay motivated by keeping our eyes on the goal. What helps you to overcome your challenges is to remember that they are helping you grow. When you remember the many benefits that come through this process, you can stay motivated to keep going.

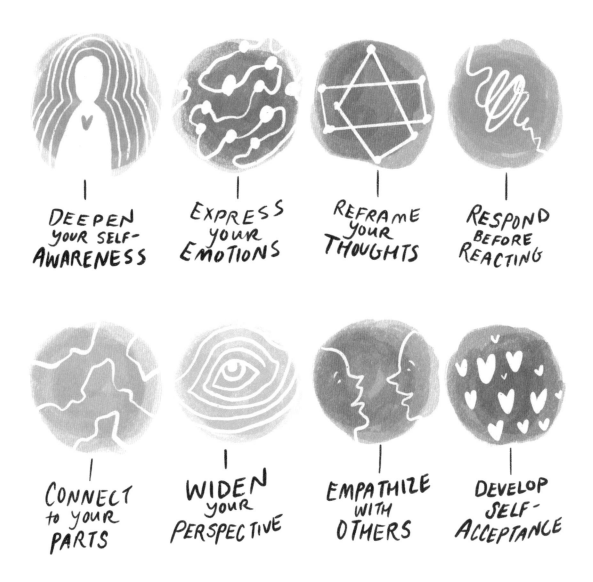

DEEPEN YOUR SELF-AWARENESS

EXPRESS YOUR EMOTIONS

REFRAME YOUR THOUGHTS

RESPOND BEFORE REACTING

CONNECT to your PARTS

WIDEN YOUR PERSPECTIVE

EMPATHIZE WITH OTHERS

DEVELOP SELF-ACCEPTANCE

LET'S GET STARTED

1. Gather Your Materials

I like to encourage low-cost, simple art materials, especially if you are new to this. But I can also suggest the following supplies: colored pencils • markers • watercolor paints • crayons • pens • pencils

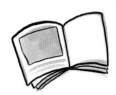

2. Create a Companion Sketchbook

Although it's optional for you to keep a separate sketchbook, if you are some-one who likes to use paints and markers, and take up more space when drawing and coloring, then I highly suggest purchasing a watercolor or mixed-media sketchbook of your liking to use.

3. Make Pockets of Time

A common pitfall when starting is that we get excited in the first week and power through a lot of exercises, but then lose our momentum and drop the practice entirely. A more effective strategy is to schedule pockets of time throughout your week to go through this book. You will be surprised at what you can do in 15 minutes each day!

4. Carve Out Your Space

If you struggle with time management, I recommend trying space management. Find and create a space in your home or office that encourages you to reflect and create. Personalize your space by lighting a few candles, and keep your art supplies and journal handy.

Note: You may not be able to use all your art supplies directly in the book. Some inks and paints may bleed through the pages. In that case, try the exercise in your sketchbook.

THINGS TO KEEP IN MIND

It's less about *what* you make, and more about *how* you make it.

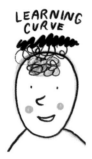

Be a Beginner

As you try to draw your emotions, you may be frustrated by your technical abilities. You may say in exasperation, "This looks like a five-year-old drew it!" My suggestion is to embrace your inner five-year-old and express yourself without comparison. Shift your attitude to a *beginner's mindset* and free yourself of your own expectations.

Enjoy the Process

You can't always control how something will look, but you can control your sincerity when trying. Pay attention to what's going on **inside** of you as you are putting pen to paper. Let go of the results of your art and pay attention to how you **feel** when you're creating.

Cultivate Self-Compassion

In this journey, you will see different parts of yourself: your shadows, your past history, your negative beliefs, your relationships, etc. Be kind and gentle to yourself as you go through this process. Self-compassion is the key to understanding yourself on a whole new level.

Note: *If you want to make the most of this book, it's recommended that you follow through each chapter sequentially, even if you don't complete all the exercises. The book is designed to be followed chronologically, in order to give you all the skills needed.*

BEGIN WITH YOUR INTENTION

What would you like to receive from this workbook?

Example: personal growth, creative confidence, emotional awareness, self-compassion, etc.

What would this look in your daily life?

Example: I set 30 minutes each week to meet with a friend and do a few exercises together.

What challenges may come up for you in this practice?

How would you like to FEEL as you complete this workbook?

Example: I want to feel confident, free, creative, and joyful.

1

EMOTIONS
AS VISUAL ART

creating a visual and emotional
LANGUAGE

We make sense of our experiences through language. In order to make sense of your emotions, you will need a robust emotional vocabulary to help you understand your feelings and communicate your needs or ask for support.

In order to draw your feelings, you will need a visual vocabulary as well. Even if you haven't picked up a paintbrush or you find drawing intimidating, you can still easily learn the basic visual language needed to express your emotions on paper.

In this first section, you will learn the basics: **line, pattern, shape, color, and scale.** These simple skills will build your visual vocabulary and help set the foundations for your journey inward.

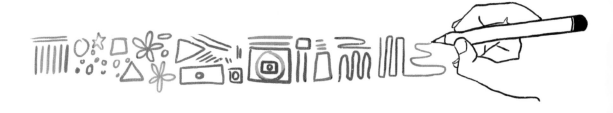

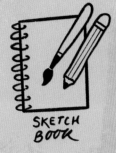

TAKE IT TO YOUR SKETCHBOOK: The exercises within this book are designed for you to draw and color directly on the pages. However, although you don't *need* to have a sketchbook, I would recommend keeping one if you are looking to:

- Take up more space on the paper
- Try out various art materials, like paint and ink
- Further your exploration of each exercise
- Keep this book in pristine condition (but really, don't do that)
- Show off your cool new sketchbook to your friends (yes, do that)

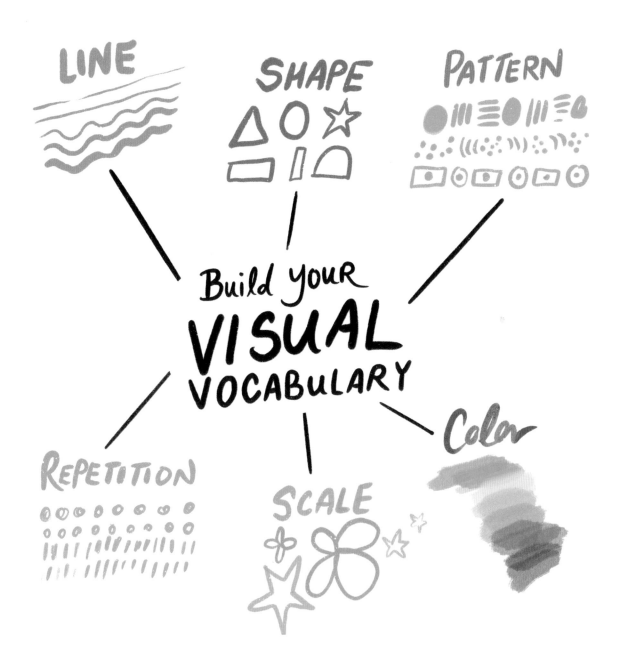

Every word is made up of individual letters. Similarly, every image and work of art is created by individual visual elements. By becoming familiar with these visual elements, we can then combine them together to create our own visual language and tell our own stories.

Quick Self Check-In

We are going to start off this chapter with a few writing prompts in order to take a self-inventory of our emotions.

CIRCLE OR USE THE BLANKS TO FILL IN WHICH EMOTIONS BEST DESCRIBE HOW YOU FEEL AT THIS MOMENT:

bored	brave	content	creative	curious	distant
eager	hopeful	insecure	lonely	numb	peaceful
sad	skeptical	tired	uncomfortable	upset	vulnerable

_____ _____ _____ _____ _____ _____

Choose one or more emotions and share *why* you circled/wrote that word:

_____

_____

_____

_____

What are you most excited to learn about yourself?

_____

_____

_____

Expanding Your Emotional Vocabulary

When you give your emotions accurate names, you give yourself clarity. There is so much power in being able to expand and refine your own emotional vocabulary. In this exercise, fill in the blank spaces with different emotions for each corresponding facial expression.

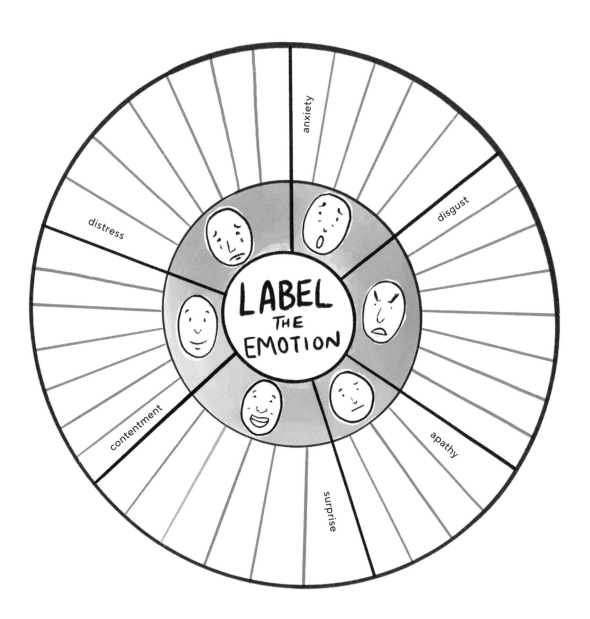

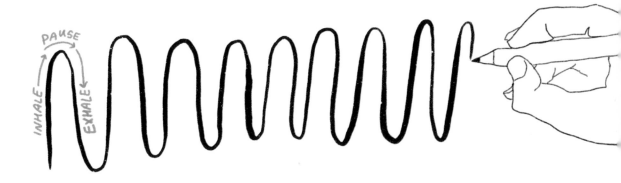

Conscious Line Drawing

You've likely doodled in a notebook before. It's often done mindlessly, or it's something you don't think much about. But with a little conscious awareness, your line drawings can be a great tool to regulate your breathing, slow down your thoughts, and mindfully connect back to yourself.

In this exercise, draw a continuous line without picking up your pen. Draw a line up with every inhale, pause, and move your pen down with each exhale. Do this for at least ten breaths.

Try it below or in your sketchbook:

PRACTICE NOTICING: Was this easy for you or did your mind wander? How can you use different materials (marker, paintbrush, crayon) to create different kinds of lines?

BONUS: Try this same exercise with your nondominant hand! Does it feel uncomfortable? Can you shake off any lingering perfectionism and simply play with it?

Emotional Shapes

Shapes are the building blocks of every image. You may know what a square or a triangle looks like, but have you ever attributed emotion to a shape? Try drawing them below:

Joyful star	**ANXIOUS** circle
CONFIDENT square	**ANGRY** line
Confused triangle	**Sad** rectangle

Seeing Your Emotional Patterns

Your emotions are patterns—they repeat in predictable ways. Knowing your patterns can be helpful in understanding what you feel and when you feel it.

Patterns are made from repeating lines and shapes. But even the simplest patterns can be used to express a more complex emotion. On the following pages, you can draw your own patterns to match certain emotions.

For each blank circle, draw a pattern that matches the emotion below. For each blank line, write the emotion that you interpret from the pattern.

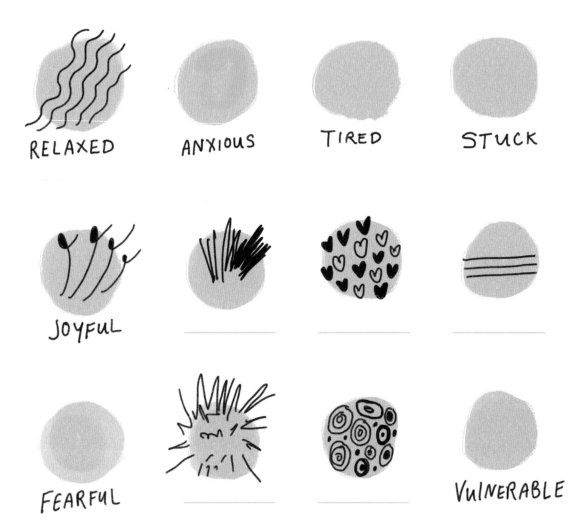

RELAXED · ANXIOUS · TIRED · STUCK

JOYFUL · _____ · _____ · _____

FEARFUL · _____ · _____ · VULNERABLE

Create Your Own Pattern Library

Draw your own patterns on each circle and label each as a particular emotion.

PRO TIP: Don't overthink this. If you don't know where to start, begin by creating repeating marks and lines. Once you do that enough, you can come back and interpret the pattern as an emotion.

25

Coloring Your Emotions

Sometimes you don't have the right words for how you are feeling. Colors have long been associated with the emotions we all carry. Interestingly enough, you have your own unique lens through which you associate colors and emotions. What colors would you associate with your own emotions?

Label each color with an emotion that you associate with it. To get you started, some have already been labeled.

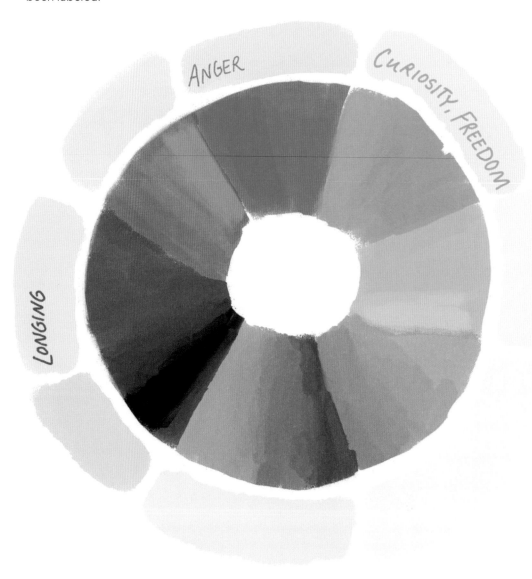

Create Your Emotional Color Wheel

Create your own color wheel by adding colors inside the circle. Label each color with the emotions you associate with it in the gray area.

TAKE IT TO YOUR SKETCHBOOK: Create a larger wheel, or draw your color spectrum as a horizontal line. Use colored pencil, crayon, watercolor paint, or any material that blends well. Reflect on what memories are associated with each of these colors.

What Is Your Color Spectrum?

The color spectrum reminds us that our emotional experience is often mixed—with a whole gradient of different emotions. Now that you have created your color wheel, you can try to mix colors together to express how you can feel multiple, and often conflicting, emotions together.

Have you ever felt fear and hope at the same time? Or nervousness and excitement? What emotions would you include in your own emotional color spectrum?

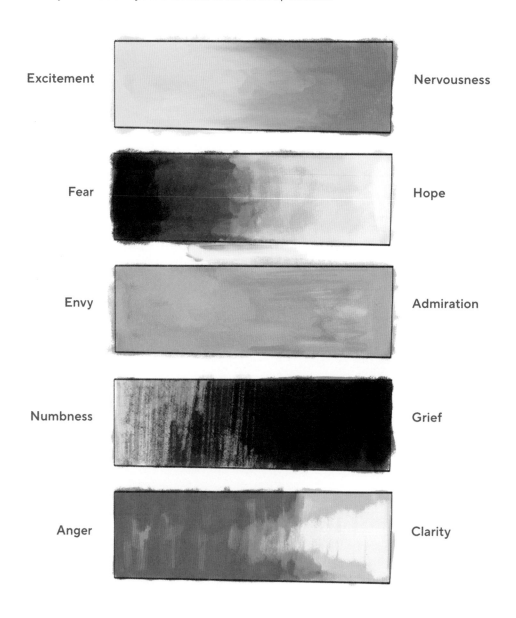

Excitement — Nervousness

Fear — Hope

Envy — Admiration

Numbness — Grief

Anger — Clarity

Write your two different emotions on either side of each rectangle. Choose the colors from your color wheel and blend them in as best as you can to create a spectrum.

Measuring Your Emotions

You can measure the intensity of an emotion by how big or small it feels (scale) and by how often you feel it (repetition). Use this principle of **scale and repetition** to draw your emotional experience. *Reference your emotional vocabulary wheel if needed on page 21.*

Instructions:

1. Recall an experience that carried a big emotion for you.
   Example: My college graduation ceremony

2. What are two or three emotions you experienced? Choose a shape to represent each emotion.
   Example: ✿ *is joy, and* ✕ *is anxiety*

3. Draw the symbols within the circle. The larger the symbol, the bigger the "size" or intensity of the emotion was for you. Label each symbol with what it represents to you.

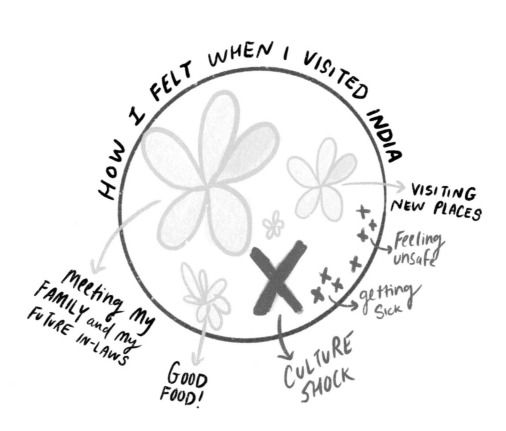

HOW I FELT WHEN I VISITED INDIA

VISITING NEW PLACES

Feeling unsafe

getting sick

meeting my FAMILY and my FuTuRE IN-LAWS

GOOD FOOD!

CULTURE SHOCK

Draw out the scale of your emotions within the circle below and label them.

Interpreting and Labeling Images as Emotions

Now that you have taken some time to understand basic visual vocabulary, you can try to interpret different images as emotions. **Remember: There is no wrong answer.** You are simply noticing the different shapes, colors, lines, and patterns and attributing a meaning to them.

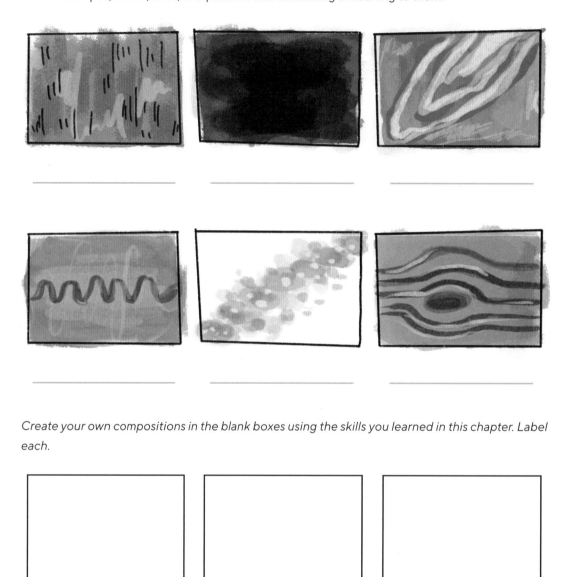

Create your own compositions in the blank boxes using the skills you learned in this chapter. Label each.

Draw Your Own Composition

Choose one of the small compositions you created on the previous page and expand on it below. Use what you learned from this chapter (line, shape, pattern, color, and scale).

TAKE IT TO YOUR SKETCHBOOK: Create your composition on the pages of your sketchbook. Try pushing out of your comfort zone by using big, bold lines and art materials that may be unfamiliar to you, like acrylic paint or oil pastels.

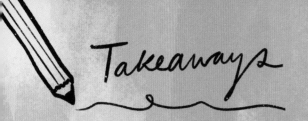

Reflect on your experience of chapter 1. What exercises stood out to you and why?

_____

_____

_____

_____

_____

_____

_____

_____

CHAPTER 1 EXERCISES

☐ Expanding Your Emotional Vocabulary

☐ Conscious Line Drawing

☐ Emotional Shapes

☐ Seeing Your Emotional Patterns

☐ Coloring Your Emotions

☐ What Is Your Color Spectrum?

☐ Measuring Your Emotions

☐ Interpreting and Labeling Images as Emotions

☐ Draw Your Own Composition

2

EMOTIONS
AS FORM

expressing emotion
THROUGH THE BODY

Everything has a form, from tiny microbes to plants, animals, and human beings. Even objects have form. The form of water changes depending on its environment. Sometimes it is liquid, ice, or gas, depending on its circumstances. But its true identity of H_2O never changes, even when it takes different forms.

Similarly, if you want to understand your identity, you must first understand the form your identity is contained within, which is the *body*.

The goal in this chapter is to find the **simplest** way to draw the emotions expressed through the body. You will learn the basics of drawing facial expression and body language. You will also use what you learned in chapter 1 to express the emotions felt *inside* the body.

Finally, you will identify and draw abstract forms as a way of expressing complex emotions and storytelling.

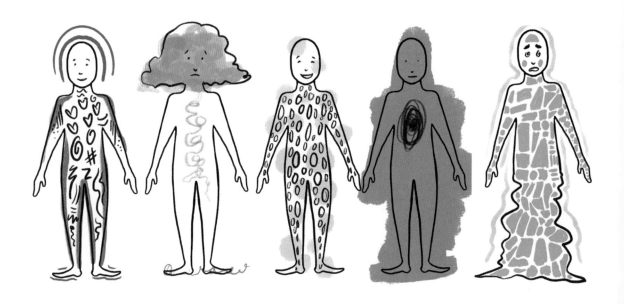

The Emotions of Your Body

Emotions are shown by how people hold their bodies—*posture and body language*. Emotions are also *physical sensations* felt throughout your body. By understanding and drawing the various ways your form communicates and feels emotions, you can better understand your mind-body connection and how the state of your mind affects your body and vice versa.

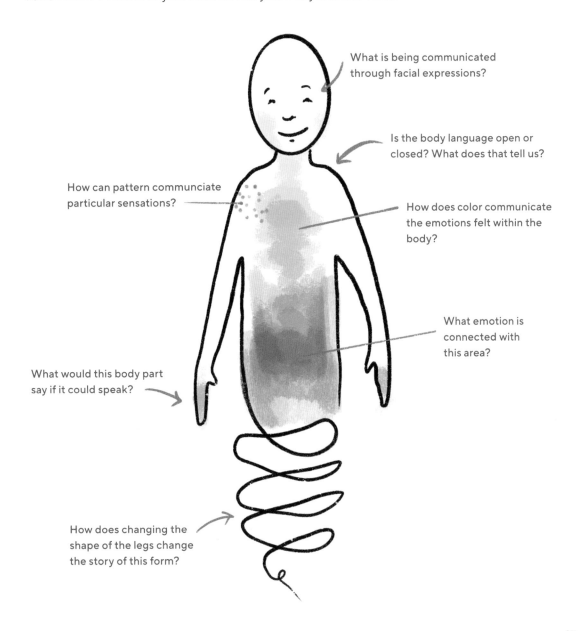

What is being communicated through facial expressions?

Is the body language open or closed? What does that tell us?

How can pattern communciate particular sensations?

How does color communicate the emotions felt within the body?

What emotion is connected with this area?

What would this body part say if it could speak?

How does changing the shape of the legs change the story of this form?

The Art of Simple Facial Expressions

As children, we quickly learned how to draw emotion in a very simple but powerful way. We understood how an upward curve meant "happy" and a downward curve meant "sad." These simple drawings aren't childish at all, but rather teach us how basic lines and shapes can communicate complex and abstract ideas and feelings.

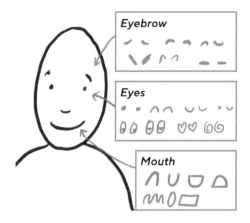

Eyebrow

So much emotion is expressed with a single eyebrow. Their direction, angle, and line quality will communicate entirely different feelings.

Eyes

The shape of our eyes can tell an entire story about how we feel, whether it's two dots, curves, lines, or any other shape used to draw eyes.

Mouth

A mouth can express much more than a frown or a smile. Different sizes of lines and shapes can communicate many kinds of expressions.

Let's begin by identifying what emotions are being shown through the following faces:

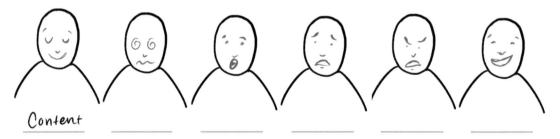

Content _____   _____   _____   _____   _____

Draw different kinds of eyebrows:

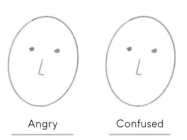

Angry   Confused

Draw different kinds of mouths to match the emotion below:

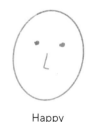
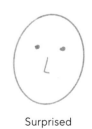
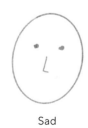

Happy   Surprised   Sad

Drawing Emotions as Expression

Combine **eyebrows + mouth** variations to communicate more nuanced emotional expressions:

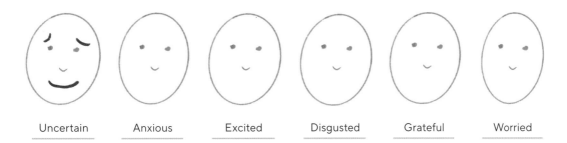

Uncertain	Anxious	Excited	Disgusted	Grateful	Worried

Combine different types of **eyebrows + mouth + eyes** to create your own expressive faces. You can reference your emotional vocabulary on page 21 to get an idea of which emotions you want to draw.

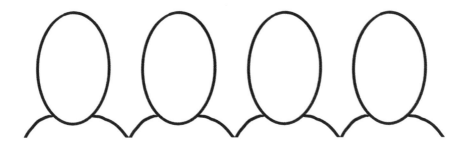

TRY DIFFERENT LINE QUALITY
You can draw the same facial expression with three different variations of line thickness and come up with three very different faces. If you draw thick, bold, and dark lines, the emotion of the face will look much more intense than if you drew it with a light pencil.

dark pencil   ballpoint pen   light pencil

Introduction to Drawing the Body

Drawing the human form can be easier than you expect if you first learn the basic shapes of the body. By practicing how to draw these simple shapes, you can become more comfortable with drawing the human body.

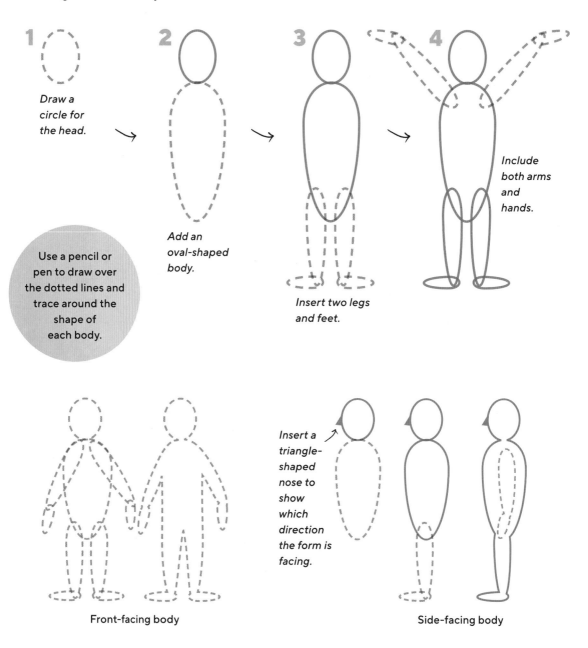

1 *Draw a circle for the head.*

Use a pencil or pen to draw over the dotted lines and trace around the shape of each body.

2 *Add an oval-shaped body.*

3 *Insert two legs and feet.*

4 *Include both arms and hands.*

Front-facing body

Insert a triangle-shaped nose to show which direction the form is facing.

Side-facing body

Your Turn: Practice Drawing the Body

Practice drawing a front-facing or side-facing body by tracing over the dotted lines and then drawing your own version next to it. Try drawing at least two or three variations.

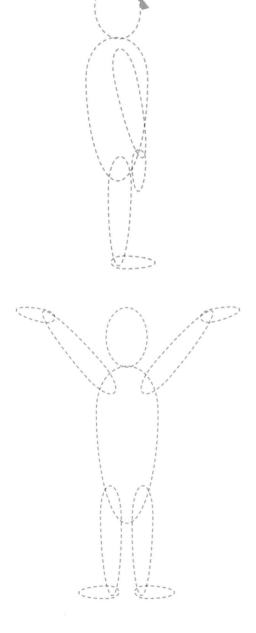

The Body Language of Emotions

Color in each body shape with a color you think best represents their body language.

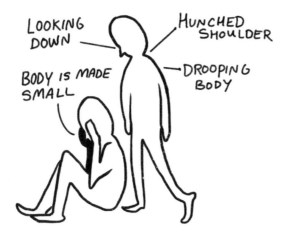

LOOKING DOWN

HUNCHED SHOULDER

BODY IS MADE SMALL

DROOPING BODY

Sadness
Body is hunched over. Often looking down. Lines are more rounded and curved.

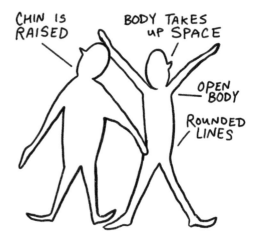

CHIN IS RAISED

BODY TAKES UP SPACE

OPEN BODY

ROUNDED LINES

Happiness
Body posture is open and inviting. Head is often lifted up. Arms are open and wide.

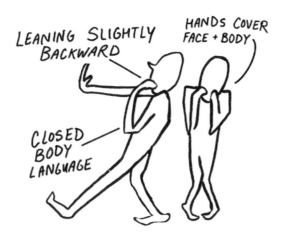

LEANING SLIGHTLY BACKWARD

HANDS COVER FACE + BODY

CLOSED BODY LANGUAGE

Fear
Body leans back, defensive body language, hands often cover face or body. Lines can be sharper and more pronounced.

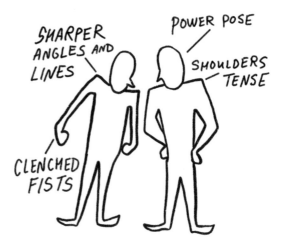

SHARPER ANGLES AND LINES

POWER POSE

SHOULDERS TENSE

CLENCHED FISTS

Anger
Shoulders are tense and close to the ears. Fists are clenched. Body is large and taking up space in a "power pose," and lines are angled and sharp.

Draw a form for each emotion: **sadness, happiness, fear,** and **anger.** Refer to the body language chart on the previous page. You can either copy the figures or use the cues to draw your own.

Sadness	Happiness
Fear	Anger

PRACTICE NOTICING: Take note of your body posture right now. Do you notice your body taking up space naturally or shrinking? What do you think this means?

Noticing Sensations within the Body

When you feel scared, your body will *show* it by its posture. It will tense up and shrink. You will also know you're scared by FEELING it in your body. Your stomach will clench, your hands will fidget, and your heart will race. Emotions and feelings live *within* your body. You can sense the way emotions feel by paying attention to your body's physical sensations.

Take a moment to pause and notice how your body feels right now, at this moment. *Where does your body feel tense? Where is it relaxed? Do your fingers feel restless? Does your belly feel heavy or light? How is your energy level?* Ask your body questions with a mood of curiosity.

DRAW A BODY MAP: On the next page, fill in the body template with colors, lines, and patterns to identify and express where you feel certain physical sensations, temperature, or tension in your body. Reference the example below.

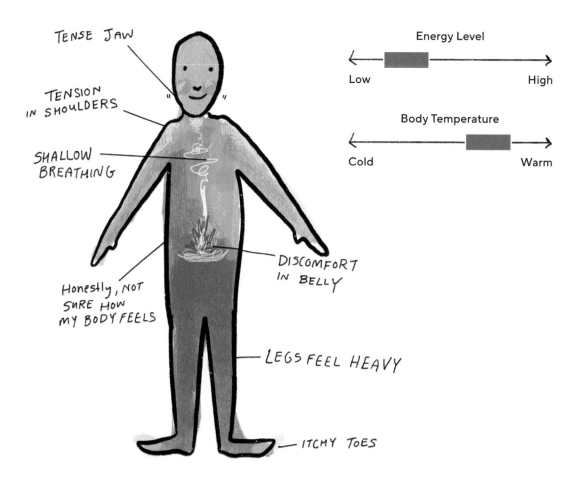

Color and draw a facial expression in your body map. Label the areas where you feel sensation, energy levels, temperature, and how relaxed or tense you are. What else are you noticing?

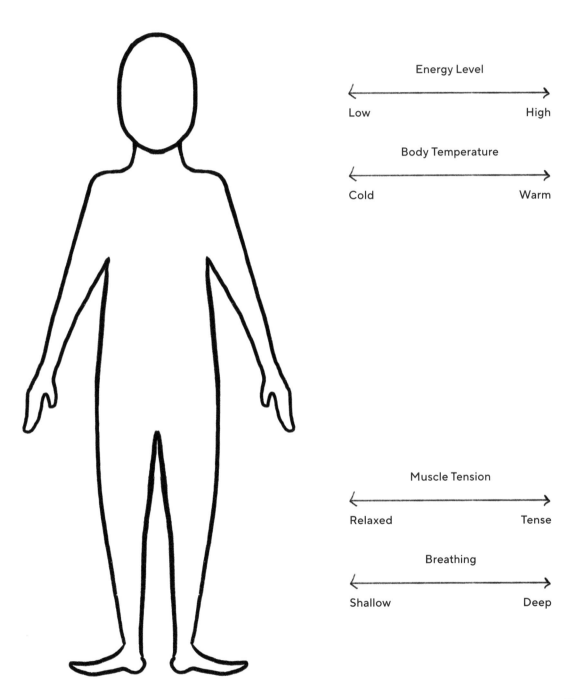

Energy Level

Low   High

Body Temperature

Cold   Warm

Muscle Tension

Relaxed   Tense

Breathing

Shallow   Deep

Emotions Are Physical Experiences

Now that we have taken a moment to tune in to our body and notice various sensations that we feel, we can reflect on the ways our body generally feels different emotions.

Emotions are rooted within your body. Feelings of embarrassment often bring heat to your neck and face. When you feel nervous, your heartbeat races and your breathing becomes irregular.

Where Do Emotions Show Up in Your Body?

You may feel emotions in certain parts of your body. For example, stress may show up in your neck, anxiety in your stomach, and sadness in your chest. Feelings of irritation can be felt as heat in your upper body. Feelings of sadness can be heaviness in your legs and shoulders. Try to tune in to your body and the way it feels emotions physically.

Below, color in the locations where you may feel certain emotions and label the bodies that are already colored in. Reference your emotional color wheel on page 27 if needed.

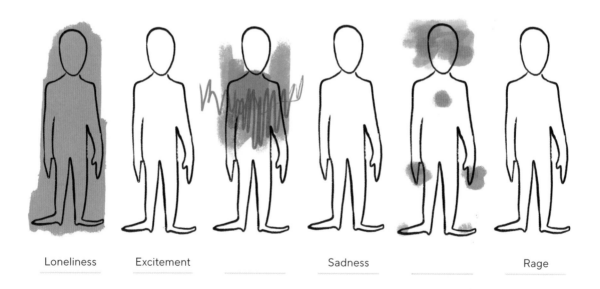

Loneliness   Excitement   Sadness   Rage

Journaling: How Does It Feel in Your Body?

1. What person/place/thing boosts your energy and how does that FEEL in your body?

   Example: Being at the beach releases tension in my shoulders; my chest expands and my breathing deepens.

2. What person/place/thing pulls down your energy and how does that FEEL in your body?

   Example: Speaking publicly makes my heart race and stomach feel heavy, and brings heat to my neck and face.

3. What particular body part would you thank if you could, and what would you say?

   Example: I thank my liver for working around the clock for me. I thank my fingernails for protecting my fingers.

Referencing the previous journaling prompt, choose two experiences of a time that an emotion either boosted you up or pulled you down and how that felt in your body. Color in the templates below where you identified the sensations within your body.

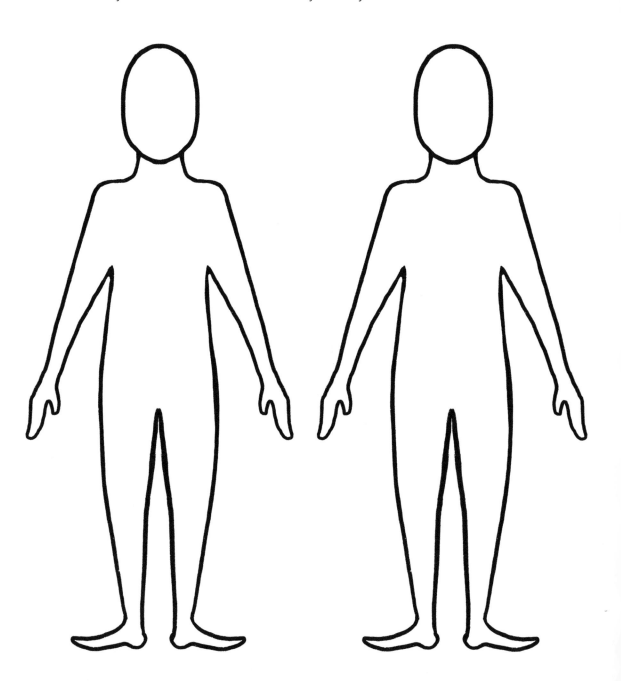

Exploring Abstract Body Forms

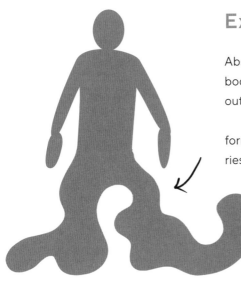

Abstract forms allow you to exaggerate certain details and body features in order to tell a story. They help you to break out of the confines of what a "regular" form should look like.

In this section, practice combining irregular shapes and forms together to create expressive personalities and tell stories about complex emotion.

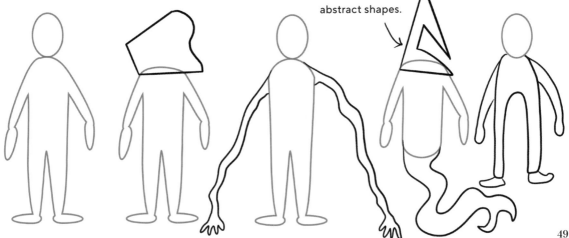

PRACTICE DRAWING IRREGULAR SHAPES
Start by drawing an irregular line. Thicken parts of the line, and color it in to create a shape.

What Is an Irregular Shape?

Irregular shapes are found in nature and have sides and angles of any length and size.

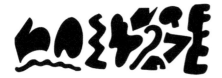

Start by substituting out one or two elements of the human form with abstract shapes.

49

Add Irregular Shapes to Each Form

Practice combining irregular shapes in each form below. Draw your own shapes into each form to complete it. You can exaggerate shapes as much as you like while trying to keep the form recognizable. Afterward, try to make meaning out of the abstract forms you created.

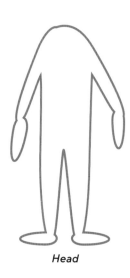

Head

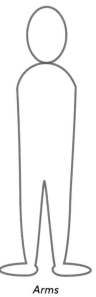

Arms

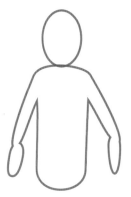

Legs

Body + Arms + Legs

Draw Your Own Abstract Form

Create your own abstract form by starting with the head. Then add the body and limbs. Don't over-think the form, and just allow yourself to have fun.

Feel free to use these prompts as a starting point to draw your own abstract form:
What if it had tentacles instead of legs? What if the arms were 20 feet long and shaped like spaghetti? What if the head were an irregularly shaped cube? What if the body had holes in it like Swiss cheese?

TAKE IT TO YOUR SKETCHBOOK: Challenge yourself to cut up different irregularly shaped pieces of paper and glue them together as a collage in your sketchbook. After completing your abstract form, ask yourself: What does this form mean to me?

Drawing Blobs as Form

The practice of finding forms within random shapes and objects helps us to think abstractly.

As children, we may have used this skill to find different objects and forms when looking up at the clouds. This skill helps us to make creative connections and stretch our imagination to find forms in all kinds of abstract objects and shapes.

Allow a form to emerge from the blue shapes by outlining each one and adding facial expressions.

BLOB SHAPES: *Try using marker to outline each blob and create an expressive form.*

Personifying Objects as Form

Personify each object below by outlining them, then adding arms, legs, and facial expressions. Have fun giving the different objects personality.

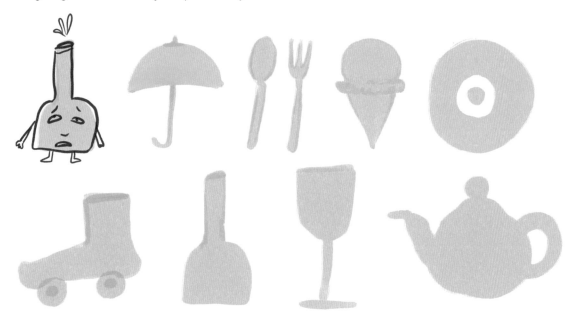

Below, draw the outline of one or two simple objects that are in front of you and personify them.

BONUS: If these objects could speak to each other, what would they say? Try adding a few speech bubbles and see what kind of dialogue emerges from your drawings.

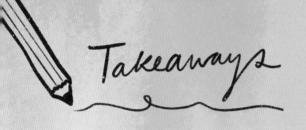
Takeaways

Reflect on your experience of chapter 2. What exercises stood out to you and why?

_____

_____

_____

_____

_____

_____

_____

_____

_____

CHAPTER 2 EXERCISES

☐ Drawing Emotions as Expression

☐ Your Turn: Practice Drawing the Body

☐ The Body Language of Emotions

☐ Noticing Sensations within the Body

☐ Where Do Emotions Show Up in Your Body?

☐ Draw Your Own Abstract Form

☐ Drawing Blobs as Form

☐ Personifying Objects as Form

3

EMOTIONS
AS METAPHOR

making the
INVISIBLE VISIBLE

Emotions are not seen or perceived through our eyes. So, how do we draw something that is invisible? We can do so by creating comparisons between two different objects, people, or things. In other words, we will use metaphors to draw our emotions.

Metaphors are small but loaded with meaning. They help you to create associations that are not linear and obvious. This is the magic that helps you unlock your creativity and turn abstract feelings into concrete images.

You will be guided on how to create and extend your metaphors through the use of symbols as well as poetry. You will build on what you learned in the previous chapters and combine metaphor with the body and other visual vocabulary.

This chapter sets the foundation for how we can take an intangible, complex feeling and turn it into a simple but powerful image that will tell a deeper story of how we feel.

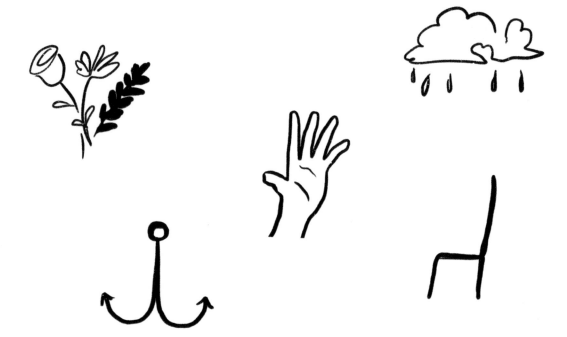

ABSTRACT
NOUNS

INTANGIBLE IDEAS THAT ARE _INVISIBLE_ TO YOUR 5 SENSES

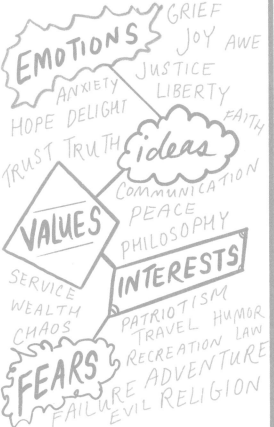

EMOTIONS — GRIEF JOY AWE

ANXIETY JUSTICE LIBERTY

HOPE DELIGHT

TRUST TRUTH — ideas

FAITH

COMMUNICATION

VALUES

PEACE

PHILOSOPHY

INTERESTS

SERVICE

WEALTH

CHAOS

PATRIOTISM

TRAVEL HUMOR

RECREATION LAW

FEARS

FAILURE ADVENTURE

EVIL RELIGION

CONCRETE
NOUNS

PERSON, PLACE, OR THING THAT CAN BE EXPERIENCED WITH YOUR 5 SENSES

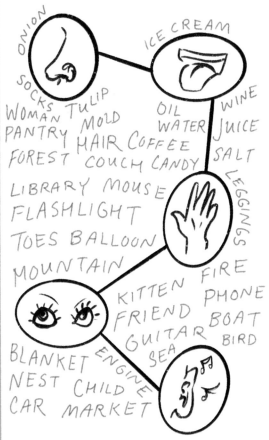

ONION

ICE CREAM

SOCKS TULIP

WOMAN MOLD OIL WINE

PANTRY WATER JUICE

HAIR COFFEE

FOREST COUCH CANDY SALT

LIBRARY MOUSE

FLASHLIGHT

TOES BALLOON

MOUNTAIN

LEGGINGS

FIRE

KITTEN PHONE

FRIEND BOAT

GUITAR BIRD

SEA

ENGINE

BLANKET

NEST CHILD

CAR MARKET

How do we draw something that we can't see? Emotions fall under the category of abstract nouns. They represent intangible ideas that are invisible to our senses. Through drawing, we can use concrete nouns as a comparison, or metaphor, in order to understand our emotions.

Emotions as Metaphor

Metaphor is a powerful way to create associations and compare something that is otherwise too abstract to understand. In this exercise, you will begin to make word associations that are not linear or obvious but will help you to define how a particular emotion feels.

Below, circle an adjective and concrete noun for each emotion. Try your best to not overthink the exercise. Allow yourself to make surprising and unlikely connections, even if they don't make sense immediately. *Feel free to reuse a word as many times as you like. No need to complete them all at once.*

EMOTION	ADJECTIVE		CONCRETE NOUN		
belonging	warm	thick	blanket	mountain	bicycle
disappointment	cold	thin	train	bedroom	hug
worry	sharp	bouncy	door	ladder	friend
loneliness	loud	quiet	lion	sea	sunshine
anger	sticky	deep	anchor	balloon	jungle
confidence	bright	bottomless	hurricane	lemon	telescope
gratitude	open	patient	poison	highway	ice cube
shame	empty	restless	kitten	soldier	flashlight
anxiety	weary	soft	ball	mitten	funeral
grief	stormy	frigid	sunflower	hole	traveler
envy	heavy	hollow	wastebin	lightning	compass
pride	large	familiar	armchair	engine	tulip
love	dense	vibrant	nest	house	party
compassion	tender	distant	pudding	sky	dining table

On the next page, write out the metaphor for each emotion. You can use words you gathered from the word bank on this page, or use your own adjectives and concrete nouns. Attribute a color and shape to each metaphor in the given column.

EMOTION	ADJECTIVE	COLOR	CONCRETE NOUN	SHAPE
Belonging is a . . .	warm		blanket	
Grief is a . . .				
Anxiety is a . . .				
Pride is a . . .				
Shame is a . . .				
Gratitude is a . . .				
Loneliness is a . . .				
Love is a . . .				

Introduction to Universal Symbols

A symbol represents an idea, concept, or feeling. It's abstract and nonrepresentational. Even basic shapes can be symbols that signify deeper meaning, like the examples below.

Circle:
cycles,
wholeness,
completion

Square:
security,
trust,
balance

Triangle:
unity,
importance,
power, stability

Heart:
love, romance,
kindness,
affection

Star:
justice,
excellence,
magic, spirituality

Shapes with hard corners and straight lines suggest stability and groundedness. Shapes with curved lines provide a sense of movement, fluidity, continuity, and informality.

A universal symbol is an image or shape that is widely recognized and understood by most people.

   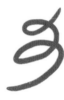 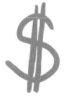

Plant:
growth

Exclamation:
importance

Arrow:
direction

Upward spiral:
transformation

Dollar sign:
money

Draw the Universal Symbols You Know

We are surrounded by symbols. The letters you are reading on this page are symbols. If you look around you right now, you will likely find many symbols.

Personal Symbols vs. Universal Symbols

While universal symbols are widely recognized and understood by most people, personal symbols are not. **Your personal symbols are defined and recognized by you.** They can be as simple or complex as you like. Your symbols are meant to represent your personal emotions and thoughts.

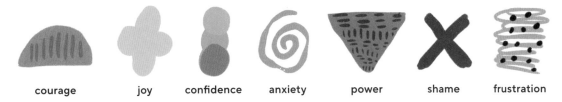

| courage | joy | confidence | anxiety | power | shame | frustration |

Practice Creating Personal Symbols

Refer to your metaphors from page 59 and draw out your symbol as a simple shape and color. You can consider adding lines, patterns, scale, and even facial expressions, but be mindful to keep it simple. It doesn't need to be recognizable or even make immediate sense to you.

WHAT'S THE DIFFERENCE BETWEEN A SYMBOL AND AN ICON?
A symbol represents something that is abstract or subjective in nature, whereas an icon is a pictorial representation of an object or product. An icon is usually immediately recognizable, whereas a symbol is open to interpretation and its meaning must be learned.

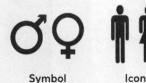

Symbol   Icon

Emotional Metaphors as Symbols

Now that you have made symbols out of simple shapes, you will unpack your emotional metaphors and practice drawing concrete nouns as symbols.

*Below each symbol is its corresponding emotional metaphor. On the **red** lines, write the emotion that matches the symbol and description. On the **blue** lines, draw the symbol as best you can.*

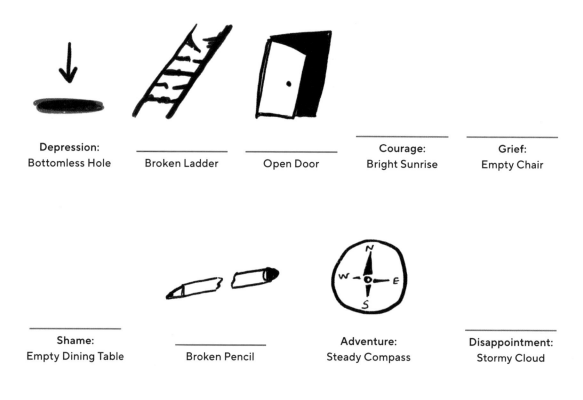

Depression:
Bottomless Hole

_____
Broken Ladder

_____
Open Door

_____
Courage:
Bright Sunrise

_____
Grief:
Empty Chair

_____
Shame:
Empty Dining Table

_____
Broken Pencil

Adventure:
Steady Compass

_____
Disappointment:
Stormy Cloud

Anxiety:
Shattered Mug

_____
Loneliness:
Deflated Balloon

_____
Hope:
Vibrant Flowers

_____
Trust:
Heavy Anchor

_____
Open Hand

Create a Symbol Library

Personal symbols help to make abstract ideas concrete. Reference your emotional metaphors on page 59 and draw out a symbol for some of them in the box below. Remember, it doesn't need to be an accurate representation. Its purpose is simply to help you make meaning of your emotions.

What Story Is Being Told?

Now that we have created a variety of personal symbols, we can get creative with how we combine them to tell different stories. We will first practice identifying the story with the following symbols:

On the blank line, write your interpretation of which emotion each symbol stands for. Then share the message or story being told with this combination of symbols.

Shattered Mug: _____

Flowers: _____

What message is being conveyed?

_____

_____

_____

Empty Chair: _____

Flowers: _____

What message is being conveyed?

_____

_____

What story do these symbols tell together?

_____

_____

_____

_____

_____

_____

_____

_____

Storytelling through Symbols

Choose two or more symbols from your symbol library that you want to combine into a larger composition. Ask yourself: What story am I telling by combining these symbols?

TAKE IT TO YOUR SKETCHBOOK: Create a composition using at least two contrasting emotions that appear to be opposites. For example: loneliness and gratitude, or anxiety and ease. Challenge yourself to take up one or more pages to draw the composition.

Extending the Metaphor through Poetry

1. Referencing your emotional metaphors on page 59, choose one emotion you want to explore more deeply. For this example, I chose to explore my metaphor of confidence:

    Confidence is a patient sky

2. List out the characteristics of the concrete noun in further detail.

    Confidence is a patient sky
    Vast, expansive, clear

3. Metaphorically speaking, where can you find this concrete noun?

    Confidence is a patient sky
    Vast, expansive, clear
    It expands beyond me, giving shelter and light

4. Finally, close the poem by stating how you relate with the metaphor. What feelings come up for you in response?

    Confidence is a patient sky
    Vast, expansive, clear
    It expands beyond me, giving shelter and light
    It makes me want to rise higher and higher

    Example 2:

    Hope is a vibrant flower bouquet
    Delicate, beautiful, and precious
    I find them in the darkest corners of my house
    It gives me faith for brighter days

Write your feelings poem below:

_____

_____

_____

_____

_____

Draw a Visual Metaphor

Translate your feelings poem into a visual metaphor. First, draw out the subject of the poem (concrete noun). Then, use color, lines, shapes, and patterns to add further detail and bring your image to life.

Personal Metaphors

Metaphors are a powerful way to create meaning through comparison. You can use them as a tool to unpack your identity and better express who you are. When comparing yourself to a specific type of food, you may make unexpected and creative associations about yourself that you otherwise couldn't have.

IF YOU WERE A . . .	WHAT WOULD YOU BE?	WHY?
Flower		
Color		
Flavor		
Season		
Landscape		
Household Item		
Country		
Instrument		

Draw Your Personal Metaphors

Using what we learned in previous exercises, create one or more symbols to communicate your personal metaphors. You can use the categories on the previous page or create your own.

Relational Metaphors

You can also use metaphor to tell a story by showing how a person interacts with different objects. This can also be considered an *orientation metaphor*, in which concepts are spatially related to each other (up/down/behind/inside, etc.).

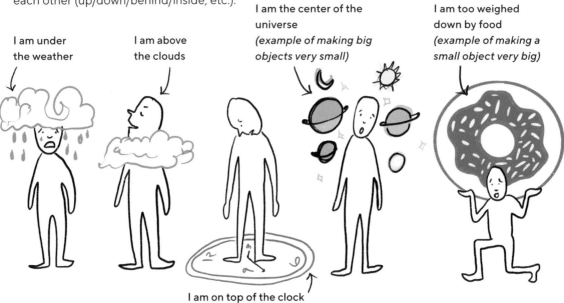

I am under the weather

I am above the clouds

I am the center of the universe
(example of making big objects very small)

I am too weighed down by food
(example of making a small object very big)

I am on top of the clock

The examples above show different ways a person can interact with other symbols and objects. **The relationship between body and object creates a metaphor.** Referencing the word bank below, fill in the text blanks with a preposition, adjective, and object to create your own story.

Size Adjective:	small	long	tiny	gigantic	immense	short	little	wide
Preposition:	behind	above	on	below	in front of	between	next to	inside

I am ___underneath___ the ___colossal___ ___microwave___ .
     Preposition   Adjective   Object

I am _____ the _____ _____ .
     Preposition   Adjective   Object

I am _____ the _____ _____ .
     Preposition   Adjective   Object

I am _____ the _____ _____ .
     Preposition   Adjective   Object

Draw Your Relational Metaphor

Choose one of the relational metaphors you created on the previous page and draw it. Reference how to draw a body from chapter 2 and show its interaction with the object. *Remember: You can play with size, color, line quality, expression, and body language.*

REFLECTION: What does the object in your metaphor represent to you, and what story does this metaphor tell you about yourself? Reflect on and unpack its meaning.

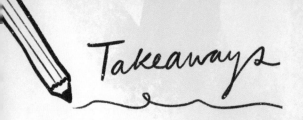
Takeaways

Reflect on your experience of chapter 3. What exercises stood out to you and why?

_____

_____

_____

_____

_____

_____

_____

_____

_____

_____

CHAPTER 3 EXERCISES

☐ Emotions as Metaphor

☐ Emotional Metaphors as Symbols

☐ Create a Symbol Library

☐ Storytelling through Symbols

☐ Extending the Metaphor through Poetry

☐ Draw a Visual Metaphor

☐ Draw Your Personal Metaphors

☐ Draw Your Relational Metaphor

4

EMOTIONS
AS DATA

making meaning
OUT OF OUR DATA

What do emotions and data have in common? Both offer us information. Our feelings tell us what we like and don't like, what is bothering us, and what our needs are. Data does the same.

In short, data offers us facts and statistics. Facts help us embrace the reality of our lives. "This is what I look like," "This is what happened," "This is my family"; these are all personal facts.

Statistics help us make meaning from facts by finding patterns and identifying correlations. We take it a step further by expressing these patterns and correlations as visual art. Now, we can translate information about who we are into graphs, pie charts, scatterplots, and more.

In this chapter, you will be introduced to yourself. You will begin to unpack different facets of your personality, interests, history, and past influences—all as visual data.

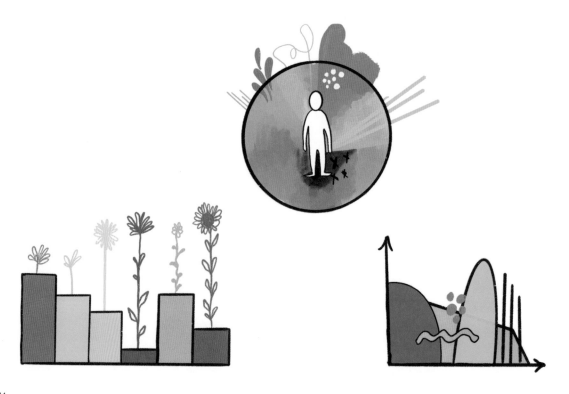

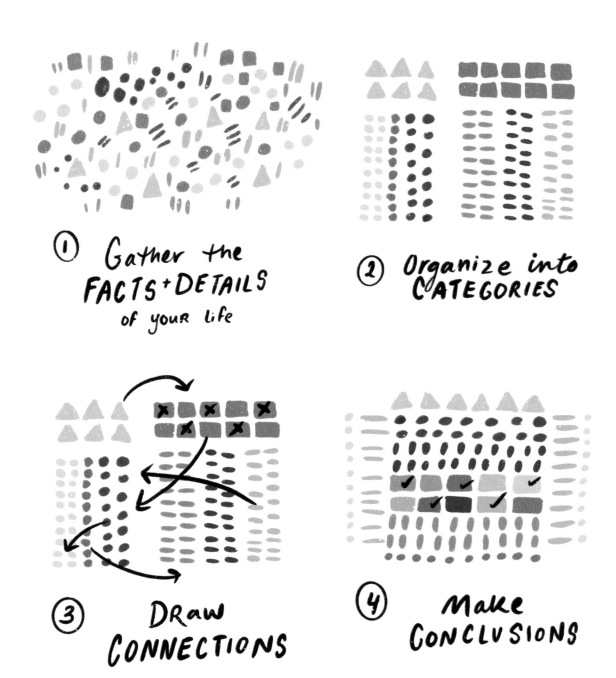

① **Gather the FACTS + DETAILS** of your life

② **Organize into CATEGORIES**

③ **Draw CONNECTIONS**

④ **Make CONCLUSIONS**

The details of your life are your data. How many pets you have, where you have lived, what habits you have cultivated, the size of your family, what types of clothes you buy . . . the list is endless! These details—when categorized, analyzed, and evaluated—tell a story of who you are and the life you have lived.

Measuring Life Satisfaction

Let's begin by taking an inventory of your life—and how satisfied you feel in different areas. In this exercise, you will turn subjective feelings (satisfaction) into measurable statistics.

For each category below, rate the level of satisfaction you currently feel on a scale of 1 to 10. Take only a few seconds to answer each one, trust your gut feeling, and don't overthink it.

Relationships *(family, friends, love life, etc.)*

Career *(work, vocation, purpose, etc.)*

Money *(financial security, planning, etc.)*

Social *(connection to community)*

Mental Health *(emotions, thoughts, etc.)*

Physical Health *(eating, sleeping, exercise, etc.)*

Personal Growth *(knowledge, habits, etc.)*

_____

In my example below, I created a bar graph that shows my satisfaction for each area of life. If I scored a 4 in money, I would color four boxes. Then, I drew a simple flower that covered the remaining six boxes. These flowers of potential show me how much room for growth I have in each category.

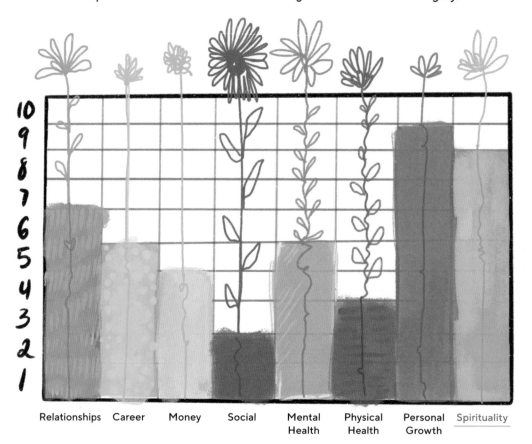

Color in the grid below to express your level of satisfaction in the corresponding life areas. Refer to chapter 1 and use color, patterns, and lines to fill the bar graph. After, draw your flowers of potential.

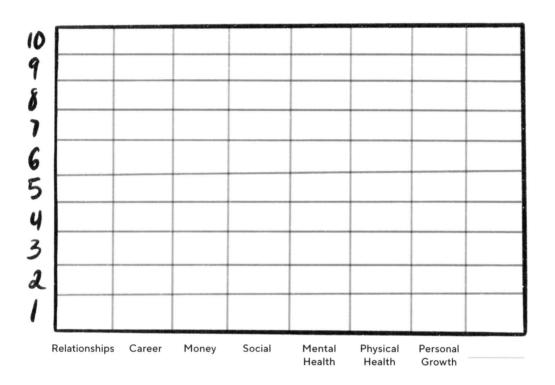

1. Choose one category you would like to unpack further. What number did you rate it?

2. Why did you choose that number?

3. What does getting a 10 in that area of your life LOOK like?

4. What is one practical step you could take to move your level of satisfaction up one point?

History of Love Interests

Recall your history of love and romantic relationships. Create a list below of whatever romantic relationships you can remember, even if it's your second-grade crush or your high school heartbreak.

_____

_____

_____

_____

_____

On the next page, create a scatterplot (like the example below) with the love interests you wrote above. Play with scale and color to show the organization and significance of certain data. The x-axis is your age, and the y-axis shows the significance of the relationships. Each heart is color-coded to match the key on the left.

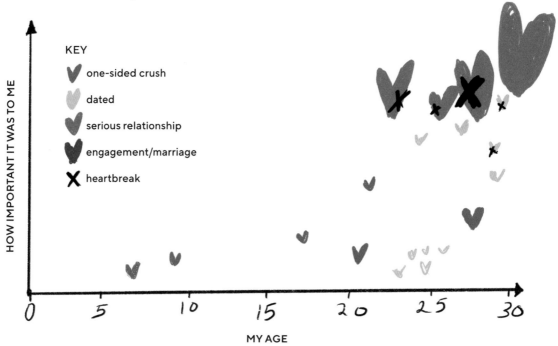

1. Did you notice any patterns in your data that stood out or surprised you?

2. Can you draw a correlation between your love interests and another aspect of your life?
    Example: The times when I was dating more are correlated to when I lived in larger cities.

3. What other conclusions can you make about yourself after analyzing your data?

Tracking Consistency Over the Years

Recognize and acknowledge what has stayed *consistent* in your life over multiple years. Brainstorm below your list of "sameness." It can be things you celebrate (staying sober!) or things that are hard (chronic illness).

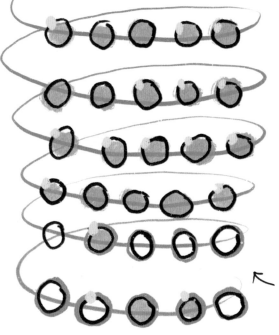

On the next page, draw a circle for each year you've been alive (28 circles = 28 years old). Yes, give it a try, even if you must draw 65+ circles!

After drawing your circles on the spiral, add color, patterns, and lines to visualize what has been consistent over the years.

CREATE A *KEY* LIKE THE ONE BELOW:

Birthdays spent with my family

Participated in #The100DayProject

Traveled to India

My example on the left helps me see that through most of my life, I have prioritized consistent time with family and my creativity.

Choose three or more things that have remained the same for you over the years of your life. Every year of your life is represented as a circle drawn on the spiral line. Color in each circle and draw a **key** that describes what the colors mean to you.

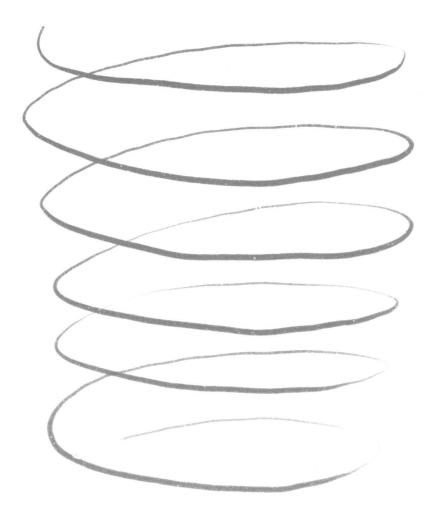

1. Did you notice any patterns in your data that stood out or surprised you?

2. What other conclusions can you make about yourself after analyzing your data?

Patterns of Yes and No

What do you currently say YES to in your life? What do you *want* to say YES to?

Write your answers in the top two quadrants. Put a green ✔ for each answer.

What do you currently say NO to in your life? What do you *want* to say NO to?

Write your answers in the bottom two quadrants. Put a red ✘ for each answer.

	CURRENTLY	WANT TO
YES		
NO		

REFLECTION: What does this graph say about you and what you agree to do? Where do you find yourself wanting to say no more? What about saying yes?

Draw Your Emotional Timeline

When we think of the past year, we often remember everything we *did*, not what we *felt*. In this exercise, you will recall various emotions you felt in the past year and color them in on the timeline. Label parts of your timeline to recall what happened and what emotion you felt.

My example below shows how any one month held multiple emotions: There was consistent sadness throughout, but that didn't stop the tremendous joy I experienced at the same time.

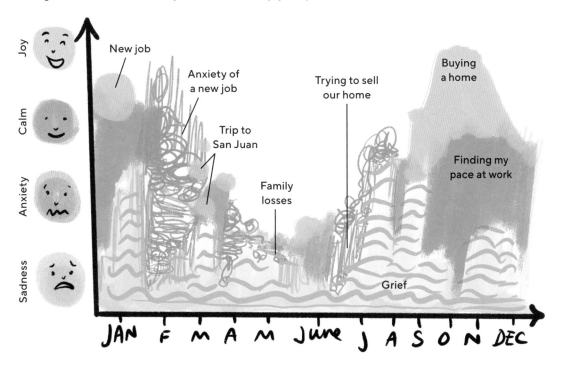

Before you create your timeline, take a few minutes to list out some major events and experiences you had in the past year below. Next to each memory, write the emotions you felt:

Draw and color in your emotional timeline below. Label the months of the year on the x-axis. Label emotions ranging from very happy to very sad on the y-axis. You can define the emotions with words or facial expressions like on the example on the previous page.

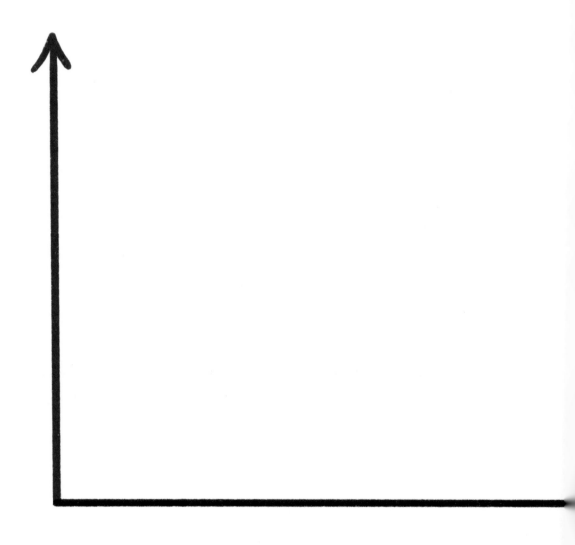

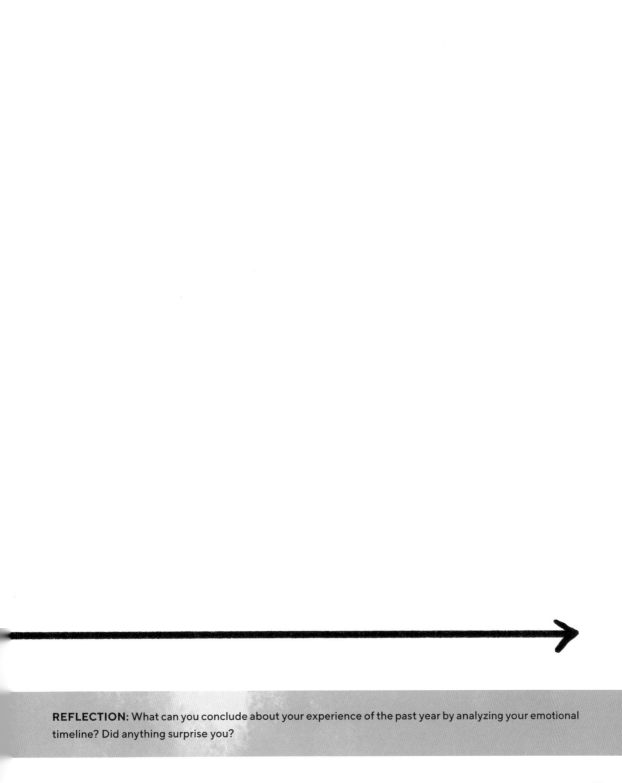

REFLECTION: What can you conclude about your experience of the past year by analyzing your emotional timeline? Did anything surprise you?

Writing Exploration: I Am Shaped By

Fill in the blank spaces of the written template below as you explore what has influenced you.

I am shaped by the memory of _____ (a happy memory)

I am _____ (describe the memory in three words)

I am shaped by _____ (a plant, tree, or natural object from the past)

I am _____ (describe the natural object in three words)

I am shaped by _____ (a meaningful ritual or family tradition)

By the love of _____ (two family or ancestor names)

From their _____ (two family traits/tendencies)

I am shaped by the belief that _____ (something you believe in)

By the weight of _____ (a responsibility or burden you carry)

By the fear of _____ (something you fear)

By my love for _____ (something you love)

I am shaped by the stories of _____ (stories you enjoyed)

And by the dreams of _____ (something you hope for)

I am shaped by _____ (names of fictional characters / role models)

They taught me _____ (an important lesson they gave you)

I am shaped by _____ (someone who means a lot to you)

By their _____ (two qualities of theirs you appreciate)

I am shaped by _____ (a particular moment or life event)

By the challenge of _____ (a challenge you overcame)

And the lesson of _____ (the lesson it taught you)

Collect and Categorize Your Data

Use your previous writing exercise as a source of data. Categorize the key influences that have shaped you in the boxes below. Add your own categories in the bottom two boxes.

People	Places
Life events	**Challenges**
Opportunities	**Books/music/films**

Identity Pie Chart

Your identity pie chart represents all the people, places, and experiences that have majorly influenced your life. Divide the pie chart into the categories you wrote on the previous page.

First, identify how much space each category takes up on your chart. Then, determine which colors, patterns, lines, and shapes you want to use to fill your identity pie chart.

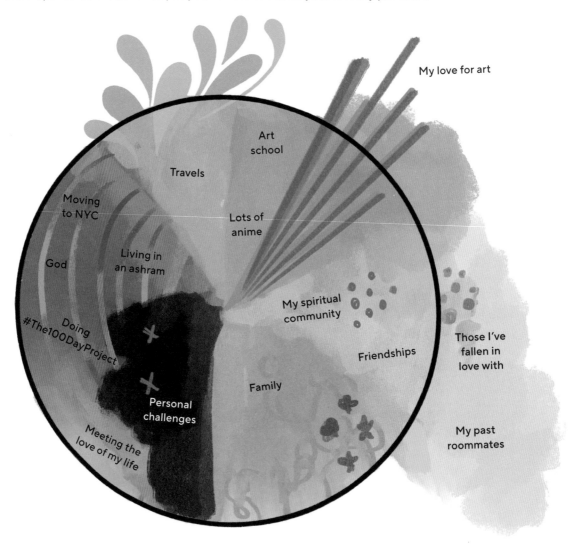

Life isn't cut into neat, compartmentalized slices, and your personal pie chart should be no different. Allow the edges of the colors to blend into one another if that feels right. Some of the colors can bleed out entirely from the circle if you want. Label the differently colored areas.

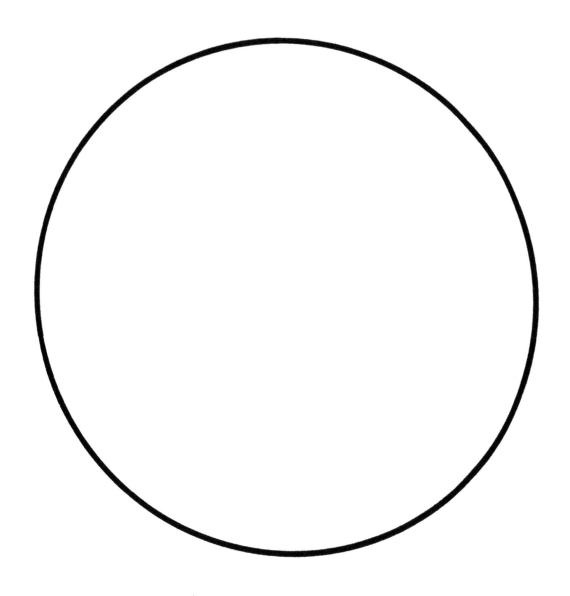

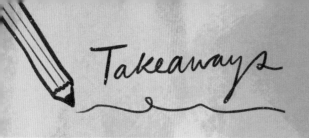

Takeaways

Reflect on your experience of chapter 4. Which exercises stood out to you and why?

CHAPTER 4 EXERCISES

☐ Measuring Life Satisfaction

☐ History of Love Interests

☐ Tracking Consistency Over the Years

☐ Patterns of Yes and No

☐ Draw Your Emotional Timeline

☐ Writing Exploration: I Am Shaped By

☐ Collect and Categorize Your Data

☐ Identity Pie Chart

5

pause

pause

Give yourself permission to S...L...O...W down.

We live in a world that rewards productivity over presence. We learn to value staying busy over staying mindful. We get so caught up in our thoughts that we don't even know what it means to live *in* our bodies.

Emotions are not productive. Emotions are not a checklist that we can go through easily. Emotions are messy, challenging, and human. We can't think our way into feeling. We can't plan our way into feeling. But we can PAUSE in order to feel.

Your body feels emotions before your mind can make sense of them. By pausing, you relax your breathing and give your nervous system a chance to regain balance. When your breathing is calm, your body becomes calm, and your mind follows. It's with a calm mind that you can create space to finally feel your feelings.

pausing

allows us

into

the

present

moment.

Mindful check-in: *Take a deep breath and allow yourself to relax in your body. How are you feeling?*

Self-regulation is

taking a **pause**

between a *feeling*

and an action.

Self-regulation is a skill that helps us remain calm under stress, manage our emotional reactions and behaviors, and respond accordingly.

We self-regulate by learning to pause and create space between our actions and our feelings.

The power of pausing gives us the opportunity to act from a place of emotional clarity and groundedness.

sometimes *pausing* looks like . . .

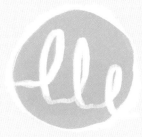

TAKING THREE
DEEP BREATHS

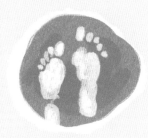

Feeling your feet
ON THE EARTH

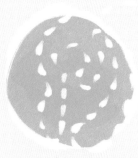

Taking a
WALK outside

Cancelling
PLANS

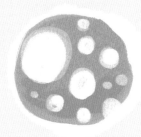

DOING things
ONE at a time

Asking Yourself
"WHY?"

Spiral Drawing Exercise

The practice of drawing spirals helps us get out of our heads and into our bodies. Draw a spiral turning inward or outward, depending on your preference. Try matching your breathing to your drawing and label it with the different thoughts going through your mind as you drew it.

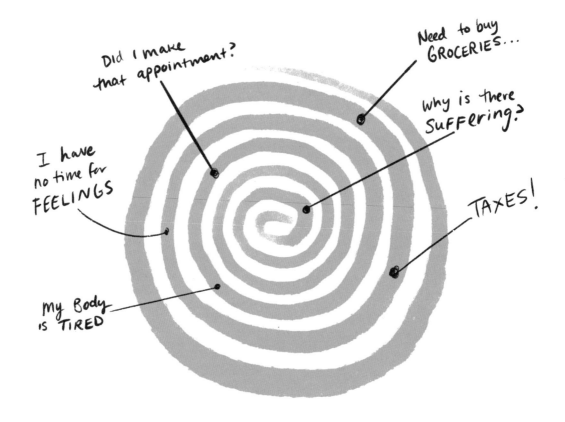

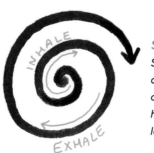

Spiraling out:
Start from the center and move outward—it will help you feel loose and open.

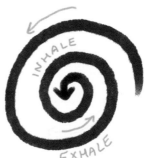

Spiraling in:
Start from the outside and move into the center—it will help you feel more focused and in control.

Draw Your Spiral

Inhale with each upper curve you draw; exhale with each lower curve. Draw your spiral as mindfully as possible while harmonizing the movement of your body and breath together.

TAKE IT TO YOUR SKETCHBOOK: Draw multiple spirals using different art materials. A pen or marker will be very precise, a paintbrush will help you loosen up and be imperfect, and colored pencils and crayons will make it more playful.

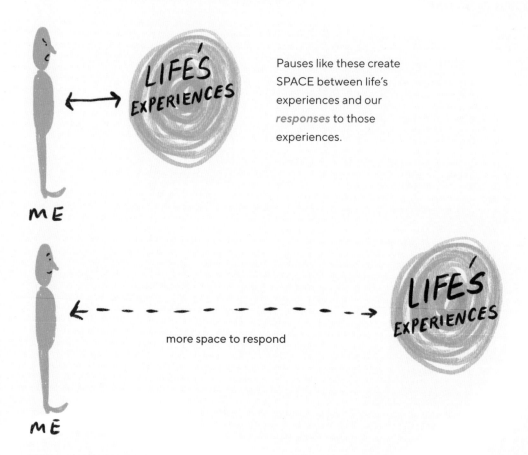

Pauses like these create SPACE between life's experiences and our *responses* to those experiences.

more space to respond

When life gets challenging or triggering, we very often react immediately. You miss your flight, or a colleague upsets you and you become angry and say something you later regret.

These emotional reactions occur when you don't have enough space between life's stimuli and your responses.

When you pause, you create space. The larger the space, the more opportunity you have to regulate your emotions and respond accordingly.

Creating space can be as simple as taking three deep breaths, going on a short walk, talking to a friend, journaling, or even drawing.

Pausing as a Practice

Guided meditation to pause and bring attention to the body

1 Begin by bringing attention to your environment; look around and know you are safe. Sit comfortably.

2 For a moment, bring your attention to your feet. Notice your feet on the ground; notice the sensations of your feet: the weight, pressure, vibration, and heat.

3 Now place a light attention on the natural rhythm of your breath. Take a few deep, long breaths within the range of what is comfortable for you.

4 With your mind resting on your breath, you may start to notice a sense of ease. You may start to notice, as you exhale fully, that there's a little bit more space. A little more presence.

5 As you stay in this space, your mind may wander. That's OK. Just bring your attention back to your breath and body.

6 After a few more deep breaths, slowly come out of this meditation space. Notice what a short pause can do. It calms the mind, balances the nervous system, and grounds us in the present moment. Pausing offers us space to check in with ourselves and remove all the mental clutter and noise.

EMBODIMENT: Repeatedly bring attention to your body and balance the tendency to "live in your head." The body senses rather than thinks, so, by allowing body sensations to be felt, you can drop into a fuller sensory palette.

Sensory Visualization

Ground yourself in the present moment by actively noticing and drawing your surroundings. Observe five things you are **seeing**, four things you can **feel**, three sounds you **hear**, two **smells**, and one thing you remember **tasting** today.

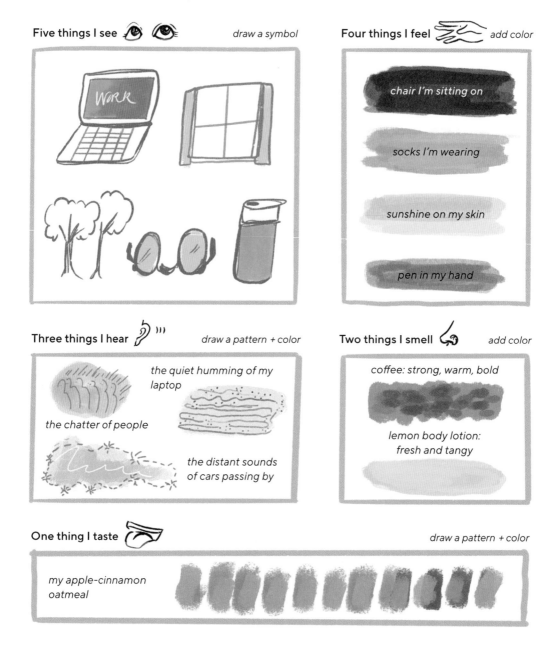

Five things I see 👀 *draw a symbol*

WORK

Four things I feel ✋ *add color*

chair I'm sitting on

socks I'm wearing

sunshine on my skin

pen in my hand

Three things I hear 🎵 *draw a pattern + color*

the quiet humming of my laptop

the chatter of people

the distant sounds of cars passing by

Two things I smell 👃 *add color*

coffee: strong, warm, bold

lemon body lotion: fresh and tangy

One thing I taste 👅 *draw a pattern + color*

my apple-cinnamon oatmeal

Tune in to your surroundings and draw out what your senses are currently experiencing. Choose a symbol for what you see, a color for what you can feel and smell, and both color + pattern for what you hear and taste.

Five things I see 👁 👁 *draw a symbol*

Four things I feel *add color*

Three things I hear *draw a pattern + color*

Two things I smell *add color*

One thing I taste *draw a pattern + color*

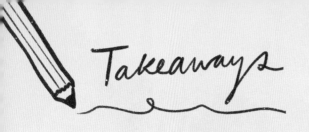
Takeaways

Reflect on your experience of chapter 5. What exercises stood out to you and why?

_____

_____

_____

_____

_____

_____

_____

_____

_____

_____

_____

_____

_____

CHAPTER 5 EXERCISES

☐ Draw Your Spiral   ☐ Sensory Visualization

6

YOUR RELATIONSHIP TO YOUR PARTS

how well do you
KNOW YOURSELF?

"I am large, I contain multitudes." This famous line from Walt Whitman begs the question: What does it mean to show up as a whole person, with all our contradictions and all our parts?

Showing up as a whole person means accepting ALL parts of yourself, not just the parts you like best. In this chapter, you will explore the many different parts of who you are and learn to visualize these parts as individual characters with their own needs, desires, and personalities.

So prepare to dive deep into your own vast and glorious inner world. Meet the different parts within you with compassion and understanding. Speak to them and hear them out. Allow yourself to develop a genuine relationship to who you are.

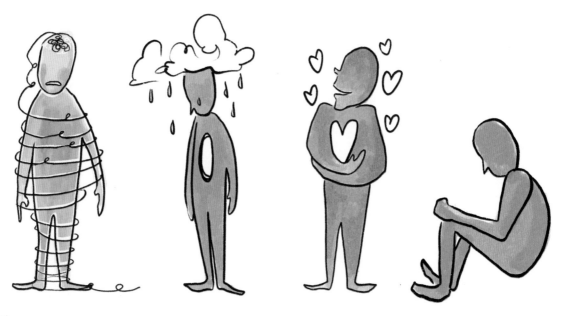

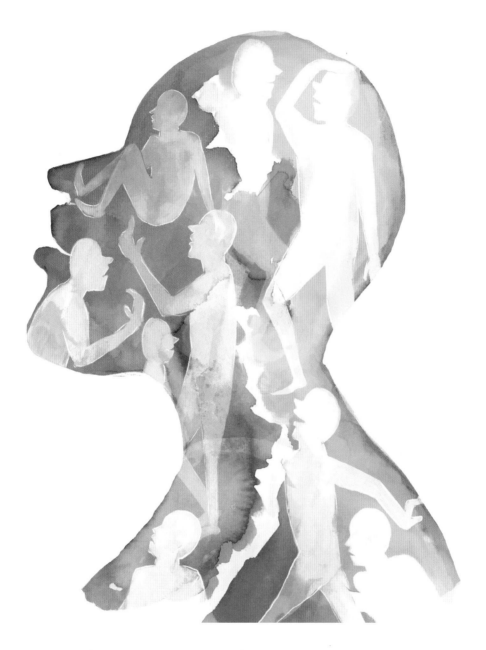

What are PARTS? Our mind is full of multiple, often contradictory, selves. These parts of us all have their own desires, wants, needs, and even personalities. You may have experienced these parts when you say, "A part of me is upset she cancelled plans, but another part of me is relieved." There are parts of us that can be fragile, strong, reckless, obedient, courageous, or anxious. Through conscious awareness, you can practice noticing these parts of yourself and even develop a connected relationship to them.

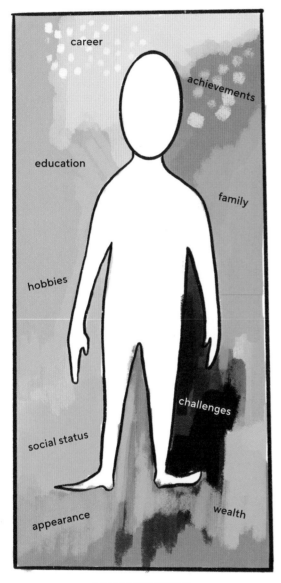

MY OUTSIDE SELF

career

achievements

education

family

hobbies

challenges

social status

appearance

wealth

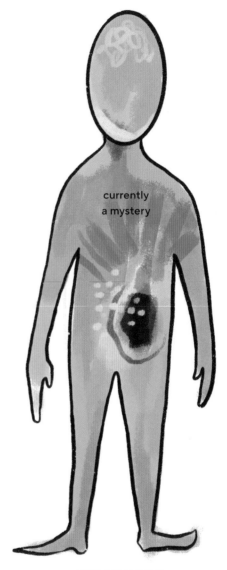

MY INSIDE SELF

currently a mystery

Your **outside self** is what others can easily see. But your **inside self** is something much more subtle and mysterious. It's hidden from others, and even sometimes from yourself. It includes your emotions, thoughts, beliefs, values, personality, and so much more.

When your **inside and outside selves** are congruent with each other, you will begin to feel at peace. The first step to finding this balance is to journey into your inner self and all that lives within you.

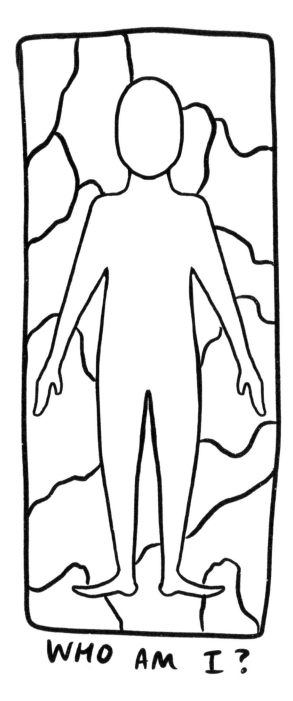

WHO AM I?

This page is contemplative. Color in the negative space around the body in any color or pattern that you like. Label the shapes or write outside of the boundaries. This page is for you to color in and simply be in the question of "Who am I?"

Introduction to Your Parts

Certain situations in life bring on various big emotions. By reflecting on your reactions to these emotions, you can better understand the "parts" living within you. This concept of your internal parts comes from the Internal Family Systems model (IFS) developed by Richard Schwartz.

The IFS model views the mind as being made of multiple parts, and underlying them is a person's core Self. Moving forward, we will use this language of "parts" to understand your own inner workings and to promote inner harmony with the many parts living within you.

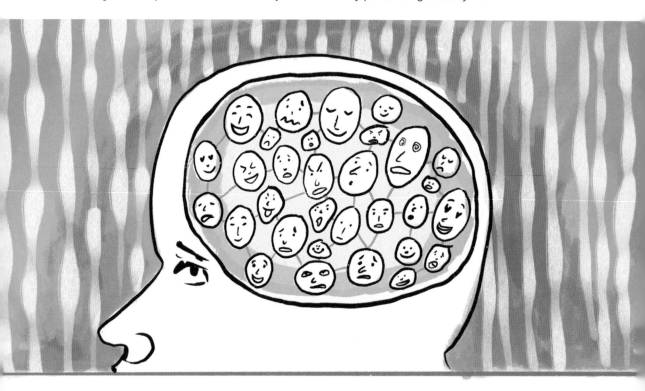

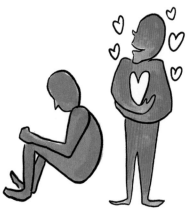

Cultivating Self-Compassion

The goal of understanding our parts is not to shame, change, or eliminate parts of ourselves we don't like. Rather, the goal is to experience all our parts and see beyond their undesirable, ugly, and even destructive behaviors. When we can learn to develop a real, connected relationship to our parts, we actively practice self-compassion.

Real self-compassion isn't just an abstract concept. It's a real, concrete practice. You can practice active self-compassion by exploring your parts through drawing and developing a relationship to them with art.

Locating Parts in the Body

Shapes, symbols, and colors can be used to express the parts of yourself that live in your body. Can you relate with the example below? Reference it to create your own self-portrait in the next exercise.

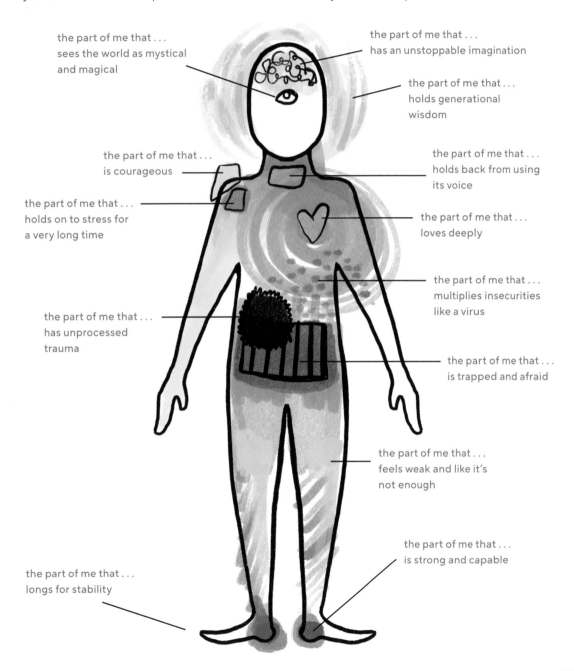

the part of me that . . .
sees the world as mystical
and magical

the part of me that . . .
has an unstoppable imagination

the part of me that . . .
holds generational
wisdom

the part of me that . . .
is courageous

the part of me that . . .
holds back from using
its voice

the part of me that . . .
holds on to stress for
a very long time

the part of me that . . .
loves deeply

the part of me that . . .
multiplies insecurities
like a virus

the part of me that . . .
has unprocessed
trauma

the part of me that . . .
is trapped and afraid

the part of me that . . .
feels weak and like it's
not enough

the part of me that . . .
is strong and capable

the part of me that . . .
longs for stability

Identifying and Naming Your Parts

Certain situations in life bring on various big emotional reactions. These reactions can activate different parts of you. Respond to the prompts below to identify and name these parts.

WRITE ABOUT A TIME YOU RECENTLY HAD A BIG EMOTION

_____

_____

_____

WHAT EMOTIONS CAME UP FOR YOU?

_____

_____

_____

IDENTIFY WHAT YOUR PARTS COULD BE

Without overthinking, try to identify the parts of yourself that you noticed felt activated by the big emotion you experienced. Write them below.

> _Example:_
> **The part of me that** . . . _becomes easily overwhelmed and feels inadequate_
> **The part of me that** . . . _becomes fiercely protective and easily angered_
> **The part of me that** . . . _has a childlike wonder and endless curiosity_

The part of me that _____

The part of me that _____

The part of me that _____

The part of me that _____

The part of me that _____

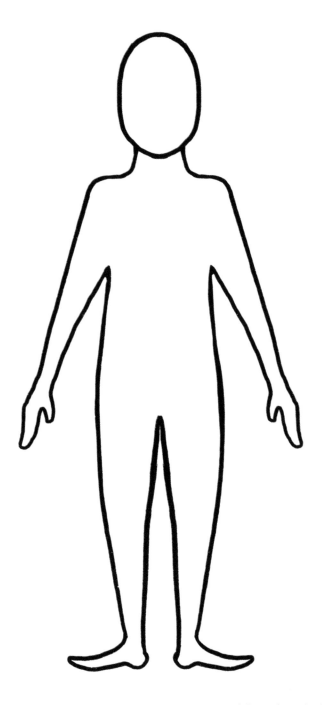

Reference the list of parts you wrote on the previous page, and draw them in the body using various shapes, symbols, and colors. You can include all the parts you wrote, or add new ones. It is up to you.

Drawing Your Parts as Pattern, Line, and Color

You can draw out even the most complex parts using basic lines, colors, and patterns. Observe the patterns below and interpret them as parts. Label each image on the blank line below.

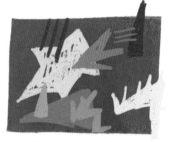

The part of me that...
has jagged, sharp edges

The part of me that...

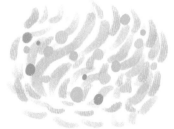

The part of me that...

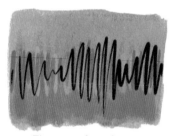

The part of me that...

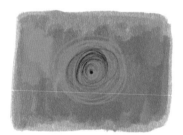

The part of me that...

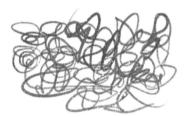

The part of me that...

Fill in the blank boxes below with various patterns, lines, and colors. Label them below as a part.

The part of me that...

The part of me that...

The part of me that...

 TAKE IT TO YOUR SKETCHBOOK: Choose one of the patterns from this page and expand it in your sketchbook to create a larger composition with more detail.

Drawing Your Parts as Shapes

Choose parts from the previous page and draw them as colored shapes in the blank boxes below.

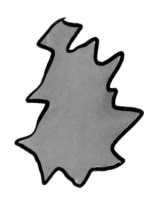

The part of me that ...
has jagged, sharp edges

The part of me that ...

The part of me that ...

Drawing Your Parts as Symbols

As explained in chapter 3, a symbol represents an idea, concept, or feeling. Choose parts from the previous page and draw them out as personal symbols in the boxes below.

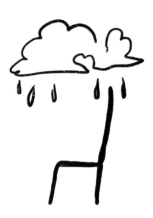

The part of me that ...
has felt lonely and grief-stricken

The part of me that ...

The part of me that ...

Getting to Know Your Parts

Now that you have become acquainted with the various parts of yourself, you can begin to go deeper. Explore the four core parts of yourself by first reflecting and then responding to the prompts below.

1. What part of yourself do you cherish and love? *The part of me that . . .*

_____

_____

_____

2. What part of yourself do you rarely, if ever, show to others? *The part of me that . . .*

_____

_____

_____

3. What part of yourself has been neglected or not given attention? *The part of me that . . .*

_____

_____

_____

4. What part of yourself are you still learning to love? *The part of me that . . .*

_____

_____

_____

Translate each of the four parts you wrote about on the previous page into abstract images.
Draw them in the boxes below. Use the skills you practiced: line, color, pattern, shape, and symbol.

1.	2.
3.	4.

REFLECTION: What did you find particularly surprising or unexpected in the process of visualizing and drawing out these four parts of yourself?

Personify Your Parts as Characters

When you personify something, you can immediately empathize with it. You can better relate and understand your parts when you draw each one with a basic form, body, and facial expression.

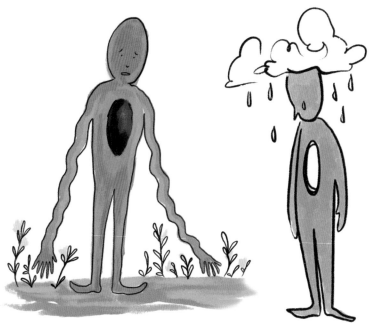

*The part of myself
that I often neglect*

*The part of myself
that I rarely show to others*

*The part of myself
that I cherish and love*

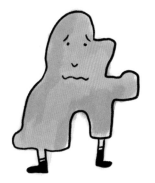

*The part of me
I'm still learning to love*

Observe the characters and reflect on the following questions: How old does the part appear to be? What color are they? What emotion are they expressing? How do they take up space and hold themselves? Are there any symbols around them?

Write your reflections and observations of the characters in the space below:

_____

_____

_____

Practice Drawing a Character Sketch

Choose one or all four of the parts you have written about and do your best to personify them as characters. Reference chapter 2 for how to draw the basics of body, posture, and expression.

1. Draw the head and choose how you want the arms and legs to be positioned.

2. Add expression to the face.

3. If you choose, add a pattern inside or outside the body.

4. Add one or multiple colors to different parts of the body.

5. If you choose, add symbols.

6. Continue to add patterns, color, shapes, and lines to the character.

Before you get started on drawing your character sketches, practice personifying your parts in the boxes below. Draw a character to match the description, or write your own on the line below. *Use the guidelines above to help you get started.*

The part of me that becomes easily anxious

Draw the part of yourself you cherish and love.

1. If this part could speak to you, what would it say?

2. What feelings and actions accompany this part?

Draw the part of yourself that you rarely, if ever, show to others.

1. If this part could speak to you, what would it say?

2. What feelings and actions accompany this part?

Draw the part of yourself that is neglected or not given attention.

1. If this part could speak to you, what would it say?

2. What feelings and actions accompany this part?

Draw the part of yourself that you are still learning to love.

1. If this part could speak to you, what would it say?

2. What feelings and actions accompany this part?

Draw the Voice of Your Parts

All of our parts are trying to tell us something, but often we don't make the space to really listen to them. On the next page, you will choose one part and draw what they are saying by using different types of speech bubbles and filling them with text.

Fill in the empty speech bubbles with your own interpretation of what this part may be saying.

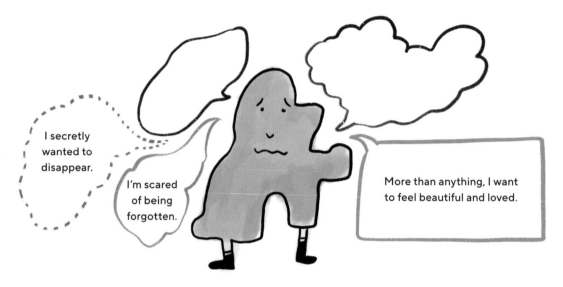

The part of me that feels awkward, misshapen, and unattractive

(Identify the part)

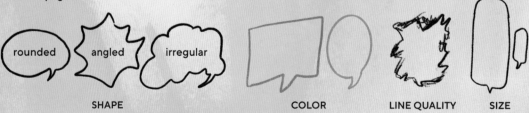

Draw speech bubbles of various sizes, shapes, and colors around the figure below. What kind of voice does it have? Is it sharp, angry, quiet, nearly invisible? Add the words you think this part wants to say in each speech bubble. Draw, color, and label the figure to represent your part.

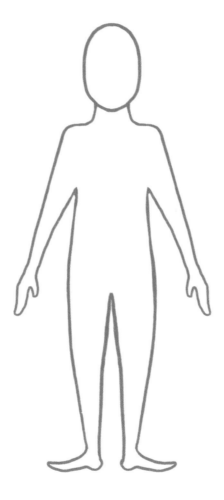

TAKE IT TO YOUR SKETCHBOOK: What would your parts say to each other? In your sketchbook, draw out two or more parts and draw what their conversation looks like by using speech bubbles and filling them with words.

Write a Letter to Your Parts

Now that you have learned to identify and listen to your parts, you can begin to empathize and understand their needs. Write a letter to the part you explored in the previous exercise, or any other part. Do your best to write from a place of compassion and curiosity.

Helpful Tips on Writing . . .

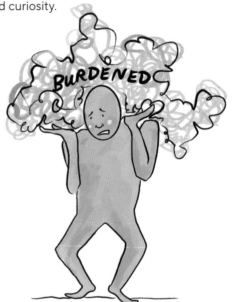

1. Start by acknowledging your part, stating that you see and hear them.

2. State what you need from this relationship.

3. Remind this part that they are valuable no matter what. Share what you appreciate.

4. If you like, sign your letter at the end by writing "Sincerely, [your name]."

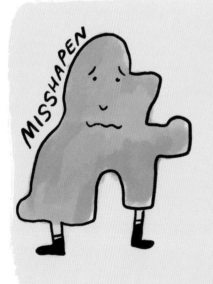

To the part of me that feels awkward, misshapen, and unattractive . . .

You are beautiful the way you are. Your awkwardness is endearing and lovable.

But I also get it. It's painful to feel like you don't belong. To compare yourself to others and feel different. Like a puzzle piece that isn't connected to anyone else. It's lonely and it's hard.

I just want to tell you I see you. I hear you. And I know you are so much more. You are beautiful, and you are enough as you are.

Be gentle with yourself as you write your letter. Remember, this is the first step, not the last, to developing an ongoing and concrete relationship with your parts.

To the part of me that feels . . .

If you feel ready, use this space to write letters to other parts.

To the part of me that feels . . .

To the part of me that feels . . .

TAKE IT TO YOUR SKETCHBOOK: Draw your part AFTER they read your letter. How have their facial expressions and body changed? How do they feel after receiving your letter?

127

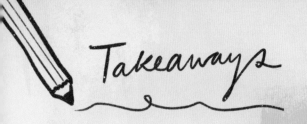

Takeaways

Reflect on your experience of chapter 6. Which exercises stood out to you and why?

_____

_____

_____

_____

_____

_____

_____

_____

_____

_____

_____

_____

CHAPTER 6 EXERCISES

☐ Who Am I?

☐ Identifying and Naming Your Parts

☐ Drawing Your Parts as Pattern, Line, and Color

☐ Drawing Your Parts as Shapes

☐ Drawing Your Parts as Symbols

☐ Getting to Know Your Parts

☐ Personify Your Parts as Characters

☐ Draw the Voice of Your Parts

☐ Write a Letter to Your Parts

7

YOUR RELATIONSHIP TO OTHERS

widen
YOUR CIRCLES

Our inner work doesn't end with just knowing ourselves. By practicing self-compassion, we can widen our circle of awareness in order to accommodate others—even those we do not yet know or understand.

Relationships are hard. Meaningful connection is a human need, and yet so often our relationships become strained and challenging.

Being in a relationship requires us to actively think beyond ourselves. To expand our limited version of reality to accommodate another's perspective, emotions, and thoughts. In short, we can no longer be concerned only with ourselves. We must begin a practice of making space for others.

We can accept others only to the degree that we accept ourselves. Thus, our relationship to others and to ourselves is closely connected. Building on the foundation of self-compassion we explored in chapter 6, we will access that compassion for others through paying attention, active inquiry, empathy, healthy boundaries, and reflecting on the relationships we have had and continue to nurture.

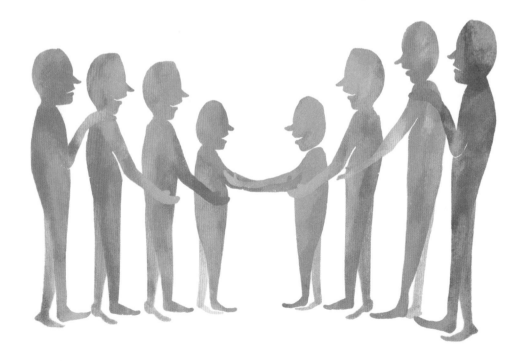

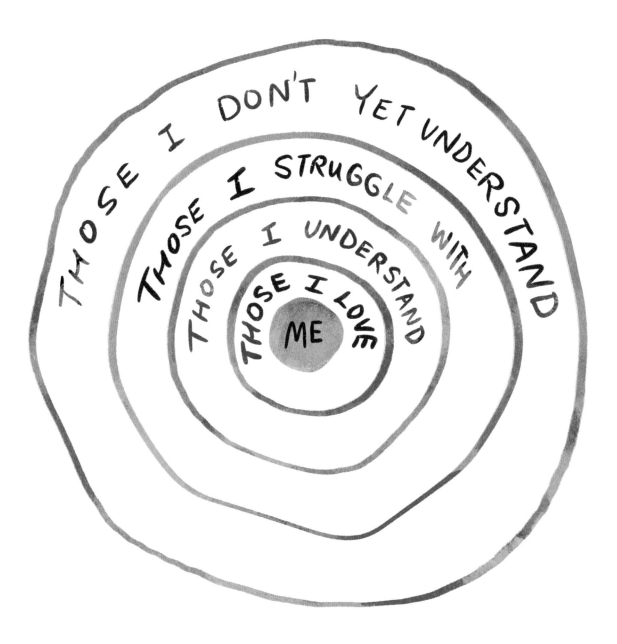

THOSE I DON'T YET UNDERSTAND
THOSE I STRUGGLE WITH
THOSE I UNDERSTAND
THOSE I LOVE
ME

We don't live in an isolated circle. Everything we do has a ripple effect and connects us to other living beings. **The question is:** *How can I widen my circle to include others? Where does my circle intersect with another's circle?* Self-awareness and empathy go hand in hand. The more we are aware of ourselves, the more we can truly meet another person with honesty, wonder, and compassion.

Friendship Pantry

What are the qualities you appreciate most in your friendships? Fill each jar with different qualities. Some jars may be filled with abstract patterns and colors and some may be filled with objects. Be as abstract or concrete as you like. Draw and color your own jars on the empty shelves.

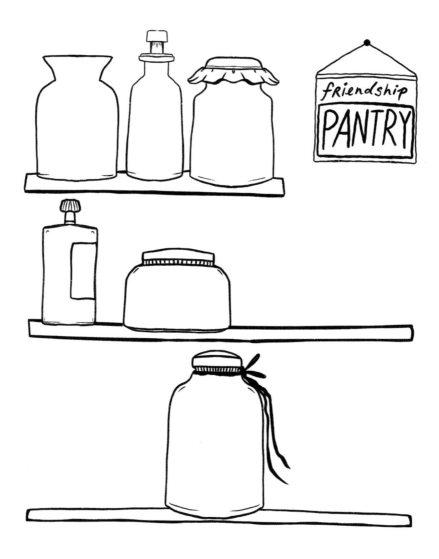

REFLECTION: Which of these qualities or jars are most meaningful to you right now and why?

Draw one large container and fill it with a quality that your friends most appreciate about *you*. What color is it? Is it liquid, solid, or neither? How large or small is it? Consider the shape of the container, and how its contents represent this quality.

TAKE IT TO YOUR SKETCHBOOK: Try drawing a pantry of qualities you appreciate in your love life. How different or similar are the ingredients?

133

The Anonymous People in Your Life

We rarely get to know the person who delivers our mail, packs our groceries, or makes our coffee. We cross paths with countless people who will remain on the periphery, background characters to our life. But what would we learn if we began to pay attention and wonder about them?

When we choose to wonder about people we don't know,
when we imagine their lives and listen for their stories,
we begin to expand the circle of those we see as part of us.

—Valerie Kaur, *See No Stranger:*
A Memoir and Manifesto of Revolutionary Love

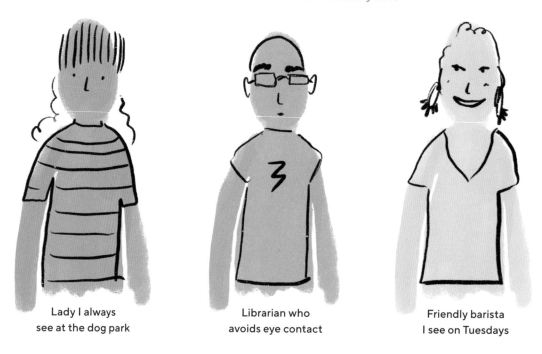

Lady I always
see at the dog park

Librarian who
avoids eye contact

Friendly barista
I see on Tuesdays

Above are three examples of people I have crossed paths with but know very little about. They are the "anonymous" people in my life. I practice connecting with them through the following steps:

1. Trying to remember a distinguishing detail of the person and drawing it out very simply.

2. Expanding my imagination by asking questions.

    Example: I wonder what's been her biggest challenge? I wonder what music she listens to when she's sad? I wonder why he became a librarian? What are his favorite books? What does he daydream about?

In this exercise, draw an "anonymous" person in your life. Who have you crossed paths with that you know barely anything about, but would like to know better?

Illustrate a distinguishing feature about this person. Do you remember the color of their eyes? What about their smile? Did they wear a specific shirt you remember? With a dark pen or marker, draw the features you remember on the figure below.

Choose a person you saw once who really struck you—at the airport, train station, post office, grocery store, dog park, a concert, etc.

1. Who are they?

2. What do you recall about them?

3. What do you wonder about them?

Acknowledging Your Assumptions

For most of us, assumptions are our automatic response. When we don't know something, we draw from our past experiences to find patterns and make sense of the world. However, assumptions limit our perceptions of others. To change our assumptions, we first must acknowledge them.

What assumptions do people generally make about you?

What questions could someone ask to better understand you?

Think of someone you recently met. Write down any assumptions you made about them:

Example: I assume someone's political beliefs when I hear a Southern accent. I assume someone is healthy if they are vegetarian. I assume someone is seeking attention if they post their selfies online.

What do you think influences your assumptions? (Is it your beliefs and experiences of race, age, gender, or social class? Is it the person's clothes, accent, or body language?)

---

1. Let go of your assumptions by asking questions. Think of someone in your life you want to know more about. Write everything you think you know about them AROUND the figure on the left.

   Example: Jason is in his thirties. Works as an electrician in Florida. Probably lived here his whole life.

2. Then, write a list of what you do not yet know WITHIN the figure's head on the right.

   Example: If Jason could live anywhere in the world, where would he want to be? What is his most cherished childhood memory? What does he listen to when he drives to work each morning?

What I think I know
(Assumptions)

What I do not yet know
(Questions)

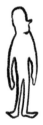

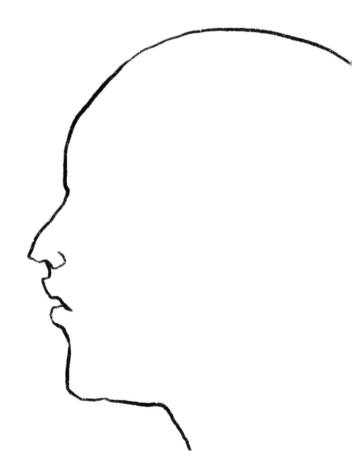

Asking Open-Ended Questions

Open-ended questions prompt a longer conversation since they start with "Why," "How," and "What if." When asked with curiosity and humility, these questions express a deep desire to understand someone and let go of previous assumptions.

Open-Ended Questions

Write your own in the blank spaces.

"How did you arrive at your understanding of that?"

"What people in your life have had the most impact on you?"

"What are the ways you are similar to and different from your parents?"

Assumptions shrink our experience of another person. But a generous, open-ended question expands our experience of them and builds bridges for meaningful connection.

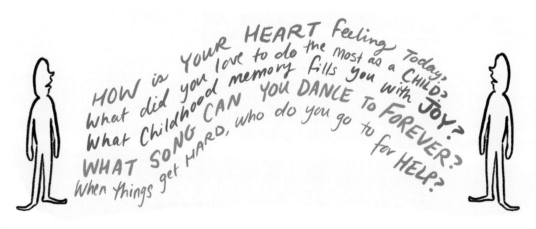

Draw a Bridge of Questions

Open-ended questions are the bridge that connects two people. Write or draw a bridge of questions that connects the two figures (representing you and another person). You can illustrate your bridge as writing, a drawing, or a combination of both.

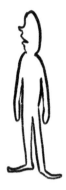

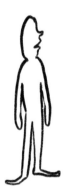

REFLECTION: Have any of the questions you wrote shifted the way you perceive this person?

Boundaries in Relationships

Boundaries aren't meant to build walls and keep people out; rather, they help fence us in. In short, healthy boundaries communicate what is OK and what's not OK. When a relationship gives space for both connection and separation, we are able to better communicate and honor our own needs.

Boundaries are flexible and change over time. In your relationships, you may have experienced having poor boundaries, overly rigid boundaries, or none at all. *Below are three boundary types:*

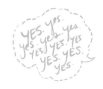 **Porous Boundaries (passive)** This person has a difficult time saying no and separating their own thoughts and opinions from others'. They may be overly involved in other people's problems and fear rejection if they don't agree or comply with others.

 Rigid Boundaries (aggressive) This person may seem closed off and unlikely to ask for help. They keep people at a distance (emotionally, physically, or otherwise) to protect themselves.

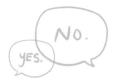 **Healthy Boundaries (assertive)** This person is comfortable saying no and communicating their needs clearly. They also know when to say yes, and they don't compromise their values for another's approval.

What people or behaviors would you categorize within the healthy, rigid, and porous zones? Brainstorm and write them out on the next page.

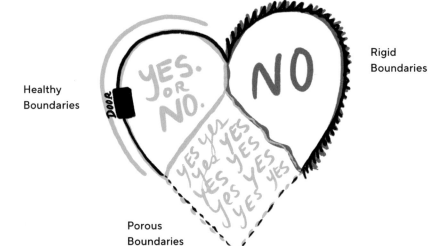

Healthy Boundaries

Rigid Boundaries

Porous Boundaries

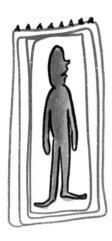

What people or behaviors do you have **RIGID** boundaries with?

When do you find yourself closed off to others and strongly saying NO?

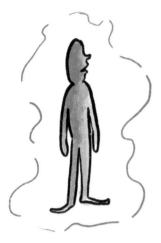

What people or behaviors do you have **_porous_** boundaries with?

When do you find yourself trying to please others and always saying YES?

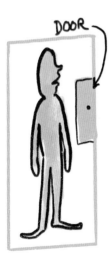

What people or behaviors do you have **healthy** boundaries with?

When do you feel comfortable asserting your needs and saying YES or NO?

Boundaries of Your Heart

Examine the boundaries that currently exist in your heart. What areas of your heart have rigid, porous, and healthy boundaries? What people, words, and behaviors do you fit in those areas?

Begin by choosing three colors to represent your boundaries. Then, use different kinds of lines and patterns to further emphasize each boundary. Examples of different lines are below:

Porous boundaries → dotted lines or dots
Rigid boundaries → spikes, bricks, knives, or jagged lines
Healthy boundaries → unbroken lines, doors, or windows that acknowledge an entrance/exit

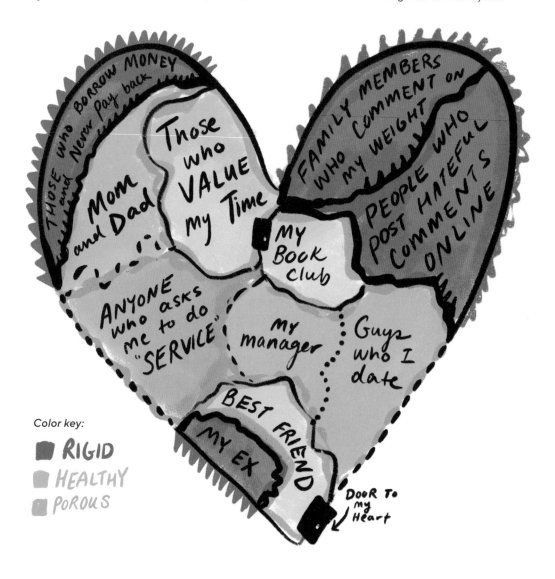

Color key:

■ RIGID
■ HEALTHY
■ POROUS

Create your own heart map by dividing the areas of the heart into three categories, or boundaries. Use colors, lines, and patterns to emphasize the different boundaries. Fill in each area with your written responses from page 141.

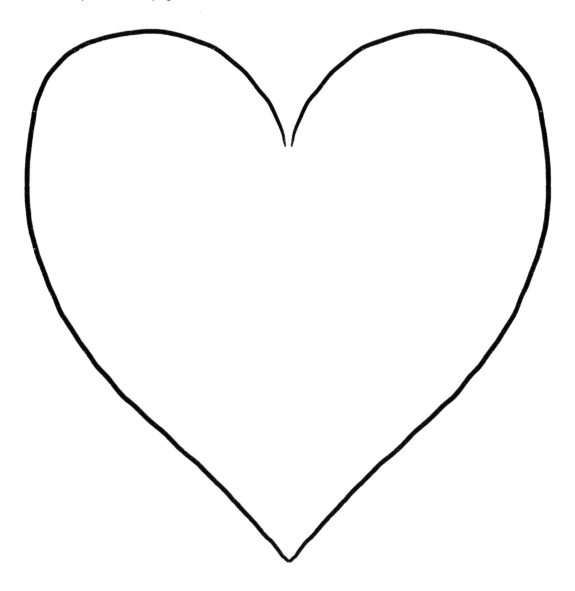

REFLECTION: What actions or behaviors cause you to keep rigid boundaries with certain people? What actions or behaviors cause you to keep porous boundaries with certain people?

Draw Your Relationship Blocks

A block is what stops the flow of connection from your heart to another person. Every relationship experiences blocks at some point. They can range from being small irritations to being huge issues. Blocks can be removed when we can first acknowledge them and take responsibility for them.

Examples of blocks and their core emotions:

I haven't seen you in a while—insecurity that I've been forgotten

You leave dishes in the sink—frustration

You're popular and admired by everyone—jealousy

You show up late EVERY time we meet—anger

You weren't there when I needed you to be—hurt

Think of a specific person. What are some common blocks you experience in your relationship with them?

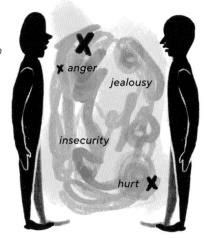

_____

_____

_____

Without overthinking, practice drawing the blocks for each relationship below. Think of a specific person, name the block that is between you both, and visualize it using simple shapes and colors.

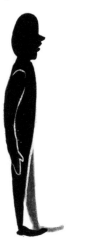 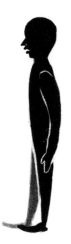   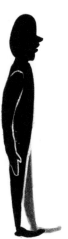 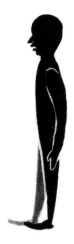

_____ _____
Someone you've lived with   *Someone you've worked with*

Think of someone you are close to but experience a relationship block with. Draw the block between the two figures using various shapes, lines, colors, symbols, or even words.

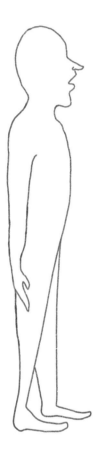

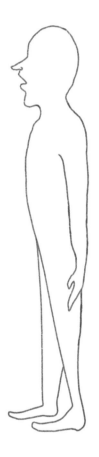

TAKE IT TO YOUR SKETCHBOOK: Continue drawing the blocks that come up in different types of relationships: family, friends, colleagues, and even strangers. What patterns do you notice emerging and why are they significant?

Empathy Connects Us

Empathy is powered by our ability to recognize our shared humanity with another person. We can truly feel for others when we see the ways we are similar. We all breathe. We have minds and emotions. We feel pain and we long for joy. These universal similarities allow for greater connection.

Seeing Similarities

Bring to mind the image of a person you want to empathize with. Maybe you have multiple blocks with them. Maybe they've crossed your boundaries. Maybe you've been hurt by them. Maybe *you* hurt *them*. Do your best to find similarities even when it's hard. Fill in the prompts below.

This person has feelings, thoughts, and emotions, just like me.

This person has sometimes felt _____, just like me.

This person has experienced physical and emotional pain and suffering, just like me.

This person fears _____, just like me.

This person has felt _____, just like me.

This person worries about _____, just like me.

This person desires _____, just like me.

This person has longed for _____, just like me.

This person is learning about _____, just like me.

This person wishes to be free from _____, just like me.

This person wishes to be _____, just like me.

If it feels natural for you, allow wishes for well-being to arise:

I wish for this person to have _____

I wish for this person to be free from _____

I wish for this person to be _____

Outline and color in the two figures below and connect them by drawing a bridge of empathy. Visualize this bridge by writing out one or more statements from the previous page. Include color, patterns, shapes, and lines if you choose.

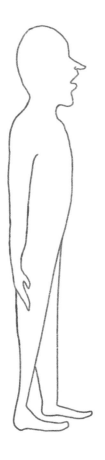

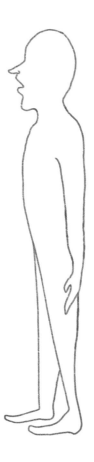

Your Personal Constellation Map

Imagine all your relationships were cast in front of you like stars in the sky. Each of these stars, planets, moons, etc. would represent different types of relationships in your life. They may be close friends and mentors, deceased well-wishers and ancestors, and even those whom you no longer speak with or see. Your constellation map has space for everyone.

The various celestial bodies and star clusters represented below symbolize different relationships.

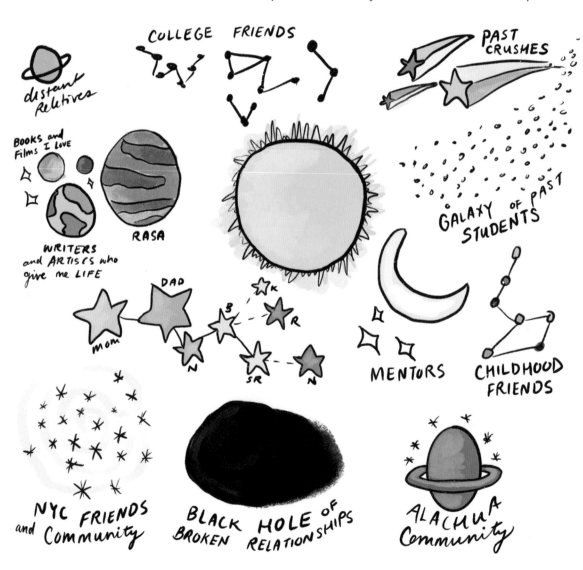

Identify what relationships are represented by each celestial body. For example, large planets may represent important people in your life. The moon may be your teachers. Star clusters are your communities. Constellations are your different friend groups, etc.

Write what each symbol means to you and the relationships that it represents on the line.

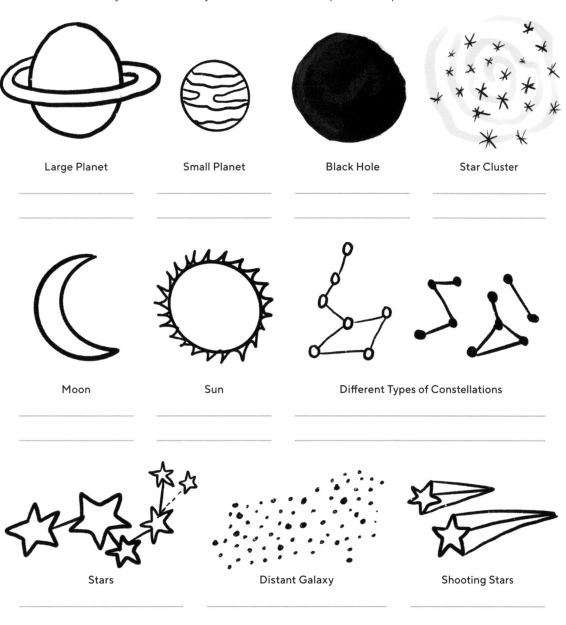

Large Planet

Small Planet

Black Hole

Star Cluster

Moon

Sun

Different Types of Constellations

Stars

Distant Galaxy

Shooting Stars

Draw Your Personal Constellation Map

Start by drawing the people in your life who are closest to you as various stars, moons, planets, shooting stars, etc. Then begin to add all other kinds of relationships: people you went to school with, those you met online, those who broke your heart, those who inspire you, etc.

Refer to your list of relationships as celestial bodies from the previous page if needed.

REFLECTION: How do you feel after mapping out your different relationships? Were there any that surprised you by making it onto your map?

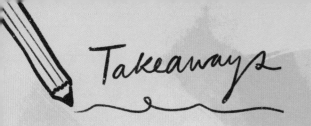
Takeaways

Reflect on your experience of chapter 7. Which exercises stood out to you and why?

_____

_____

_____

_____

_____

_____

_____

_____

_____

_____

CHAPTER 7 EXERCISES

☐ Friendship Pantry

☐ The Anonymous People in Your Life

☐ Acknowledging Your Assumptions

☐ Draw a Bridge of Questions

☐ Boundaries of Your Heart

☐ Draw Your Relationship Blocks

☐ Empathy Connects Us

☐ Your Personal Constellation Map

☐ Draw Your Personal Constellation Map

8

YOUR RELATIONSHIP TO YOUR VALUES

living your
VALUES

We always have a choice of how we want to show up in our lives, and that's defined by asking two simple questions: *What matters to you the most at this moment? Who do you want to be at this moment?* Identifying your core values is the first step to answering these questions.

It's necessary to define what's important to you before society/culture/work defines it for you. When you recognize what's most important, you can ensure that your choices and behaviors match your internal aspirations. *In short: You make your outsides match your insides.*

When you match the way you speak, act, and feel with your values, you begin to feel whole, content, and connected. When you're not acting in alignment with your values, you will often feel frustrated, restless, and discontented.

In this chapter, you will identify and explore your core values and learn how to embody them and express them in different ways.

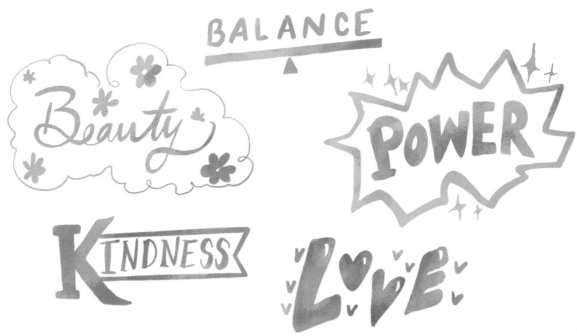

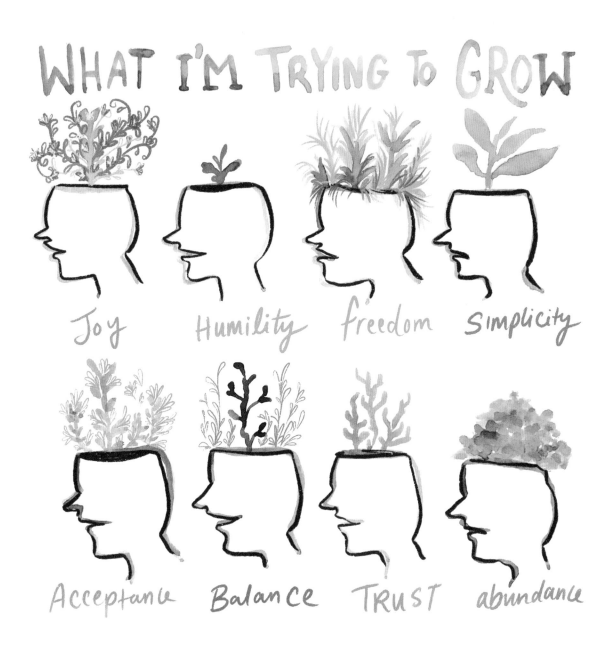

WHAT I'M TRYING TO GROW

Joy

Humility

Freedom

Simplicity

Acceptance

Balance

TRUST

abundance

You are the gardener of your heart and mind. Every moment, you have the opportunity to grow and nurture your values through your actions. When you prioritize what is most important through your behaviors and habits, you are consciously watering your values. When your values flourish, you thrive: Life feels meaningful and filled with purpose.

Identify Your Core Values

Discover what your personal values are by exploring a specific emotional experience. As you answer the prompts below, use the values list on the next page if needed.

Recall a peak moment in your life when you felt totally yourself and in your natural element. Briefly describe the details. *How long ago was it? Where were you? What were you doing? How did you feel?*

_____

_____

_____

_____

What was important about this moment for you?

_____

_____

_____

_____

What values were being expressed and felt?

Example: Feeling a deep sense of connection when I hosted a local community gathering last summer

_____

_____

List of Values

Accountability	Empathy	Kindness	Self-expression
Achievement	Environment	Leadership	Self-respect
Adaptability	Equality	Learning	Serenity
Adventure	Ethics	Legacy	Service
Ambition	Excellence	Love	Simplicity
Authenticity	Fairness	Loyalty	Spirituality
Balance	Faith	Making a difference	Sportsmanship
Beauty	Family	Mastery	Stability
Belonging	Focus	Nature	Strength
Career	Forgiveness	Openness	Success
Caring	Freedom	Optimism	Teamwork
Collaboration	Friendship	Order	Time
Commitment	Fun	Parenting	Tradition
Community	Generosity	Patience	Travel
Compassion	Grace	Peace	Trust
Competence	Growth	Perseverance	Truth
Confidence	Harmony	Power	Understanding
Connection	Health	Pride	Uniqueness
Contribution	Home	Professionalism	Vision
Cooperation	Honesty	Recognition	Vulnerability
Courage	Hope	Reliability	Wealth
Creativity	Humility	Resourcefulness	Well-being
Curiosity	Humor	Respect	Wisdom
Devotion	Independence	Responsibility	*Write yours:*
Dignity	Integrity	Risk-taking	_____
Discipline	Intuition	Safety	_____
Diversity	Joy	Security	_____
Efficiency	Justice	Self-discipline	

Scan through this extensive list of values.

1. Draw a dot next to any value that stands out and connects back to your emotional experience.
2. With a pen, circle up to five of your most important, or primary, values.
3. With another colored pen, circle five to ten of your supporting, or secondary, values.

Defining Your Values

Writing down your values will allow you to gain a sense of ownership. Referencing the previous list of values, write out all your circled values in the box below.

From your list of chosen values, circle two core primary values that matter most to you. Next, underline five to seven values that would support each of your primary values. See the example below:

FAmily Creativity Belonging integrity Courage
Community Connection Spirituality Kindness
DISCIPline Vulnerability Empathy Honesty
SERVICE Authenticity Self-Expression

List out your primary values in each blue box and nest your secondary values below them:

CONNECTION
COMMUNITY
BELONGING
FAMILY
CREATIVITY
SERVICE
KINDNESS
EMPATHY

AUTHENTICITY
INTEGRITY
COURAGE
SPIRITUALITY
HONESTY
DISCIPLINE
VULNERABILITY
SELF-EXPRESSION

Personal Values Definition

Now that you have defined your two primary values, write your *own* definition of each value and what it means to you and looks like in your life. You can use the secondary values you chose to help you write your definition. My personal values definition looks like this:

AUTHENTICITY, for me, looks like . . . *being deeply honest with who I am and therefore being OK when people don't like me. It means having the courage to express myself, my needs, and my truth.*

CONNECTION, for me, looks like . . . *acting with kindness, listening to others, engaging in service, and truly connecting to another person. Heart to heart. There is no room for BS here.*

Write your own definition of what your two primary values mean and how they show up in your life:

For me, this value looks like . . .

_____

_____

What people, places, or things do you associate with this value? Write them below:

_____

For me, this value looks like . . .

_____

_____

What people, places, or things do you associate with this value? Write them below:

_____

EXPRESSIVE Lettering

Did you know that you can express the emotion behind a certain word by writing it in a particular form? This skill is called lettering—the art of drawing out letters instead of only writing them.

Your values can also be expressed using expressive lettering. How we write our values says a lot. The color, shape, and style of the letters communicate what our values mean to us.

It's not WHAT you say, it's HOW you say it. This phrase also goes for how you write out words. You can write **POWER** or you can write *Power*. The tone of this word changes drastically depending on the color, size, style, and line quality of the word.

What are the different lettering styles below communicating? Some are playful and bubbly, some are elegant, some are modern, and others are minimal.

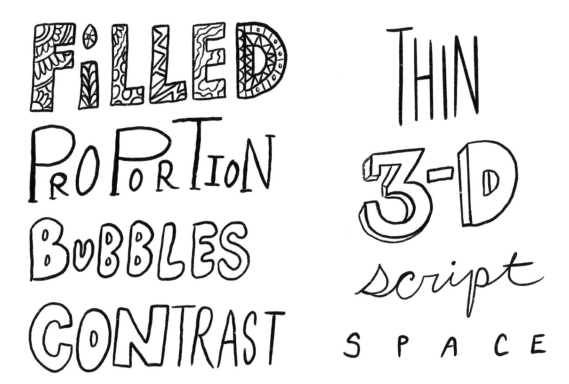

FILLED
PROPORTION
BUBBLES
CONTRAST

THIN
3-D
script
S P A C E

Note: *Don't let your handwriting stop you from creating expressive lettering. It's not about being neat or beautiful. It's about communicating emotion. You can do this with messy, raw, untidy lettering or through decorative, detailed scripts. There are endless ways to explore your lettering.*

Practice Drawing Expressive Letters

Using a marker or pen, practice drawing letters by tracing on top of the letters below.

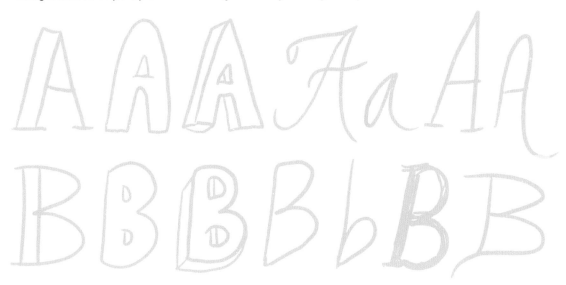

Choose one letter from the alphabet and draw it below in as many ways as you can. Use pens or markers of different thicknesses and colors to create many different variations.

TAKE IT TO YOUR SKETCHBOOK: Go BIG and draw one single letter in your sketchbook and let it fill up a whole page. Challenge yourself to fill in the letter with various patterns, shapes, lines, and colors. How much detail can you put into a single letter? Give it a try!

Express Your Values through Words

Emphasize what your personal values mean to you by drawing them out as expressive lettering. Color in the examples below and notice what each one is communicating.

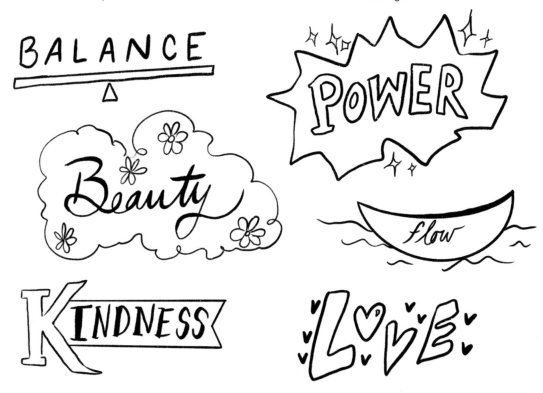

Practice drawing out the words of each value in the boxes below. Include different colors and shapes.

Growth

Freedom

Let your words be the subject of your drawing. Choose one of your values and draw it out using expressive lettering. Ask yourself the following questions to help you get started:

- What color would you use to communicate this value?
- What patterns, shapes, lines, and symbols would you add?
- What is the tone of your value (bold, whimsical, soft, quirky, elegant, minimal, funky, raw, etc.)?
- How would you draw out the letters of this word? See page 161 for examples on how to draw the letters.

REFLECTION: Analyze the tone, size, color, and quality of your image. What does it say about your value, and what meaning do you make from it?

Create Your Own Values Metaphor

As you learned in chapter 3, a metaphor is a powerful way to express abstract ideas, emotions, and values. In this exercise, you will create and draw your own metaphor using images and words.

Below, write your chosen values in the first column. Then, circle an adjective and concrete noun for each value. Allow yourself to make surprising and unlikely connections, even if they don't make sense immediately.

VALUES	ADJECTIVE			CONCRETE NOUN		
freedom	warm	open	tender	road	mountain	hug
	cold	thin	fierce	train	sea	friend
	loud	bouncy	gentle	door	highway	sunshine
	bright	quiet	glowing	lion	garden	traveler
	thick	deep	sparkling	anchor	lightning	compass
	heavy	patient	vibrant	sunflower	house	sky
	large	soft	clear	library	river	teacher
	calm	familiar	hungry			
	precious	vast	wild			

Combine the **adjective and noun** to create your metaphor. For example: Freedom is an open road.

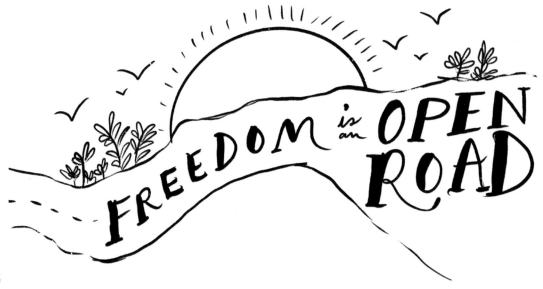

Create one metaphor for your chosen value and draw it using image and words. Ask yourself the following questions to help you get started:

- How much space do you want the words to take up on the page?
- What patterns, shapes, lines, and symbols would you add to emphasize the metaphor?
- What message is your metaphor conveying?

TAKE IT TO YOUR SKETCHBOOK: Challenge yourself to draw out your values metaphor using *only* words. You can incorporate multiple values in one image or even repeat the same value over and over again for emphasis.

Your Values Reveal Your Needs

Your core values have a way of shining a light on your needs. For example, if you value self-discipline, then you may have a need for structure and accountability in your life. In the blank spaces below, write out your needs in relation to your chosen values.

VALUE...	NEED...
Presence	The need to live life as it happens at this very moment
Belonging	The need to feel part of something larger than myself
Self-Discipline	The need for structure and accountability to myself
Adventure	The need to feel alive

Values need to be nurtured and grown, just like a garden. Using the metaphor of a garden, choose a plant that symbolically mirrors your value. The flower represents your need in relation to the value.

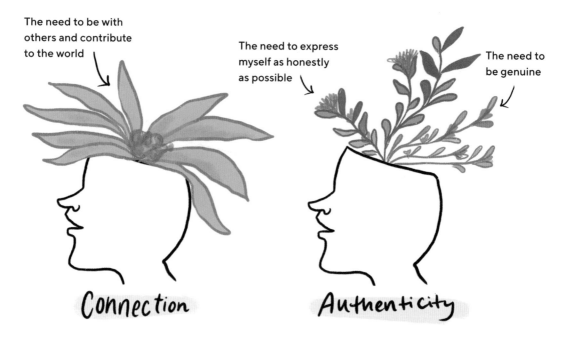

The need to be with others and contribute to the world

The need to express myself as honestly as possible

The need to be genuine

Connection

Authenticity

Draw Your Values Garden

Choose two core values and draw them as a plant, and the needs as flowers. What color is it? Does it have thorns or not? Does it have multiple flowers or just one bloom? What is the shape of the pot or container that holds it?

TAKE IT TO YOUR SKETCHBOOK: Create a collaged values garden by collecting and pasting flower petals and leaves directly into your sketchbook.

Behaviors to Support Your Values

Planting your values garden is only the first step. The next step is to reinforce your values through your choices and behavior. Draw one or more colorful arcs above your plant that represent a **specific supportive behavior** and will help to nurture and grow your value.

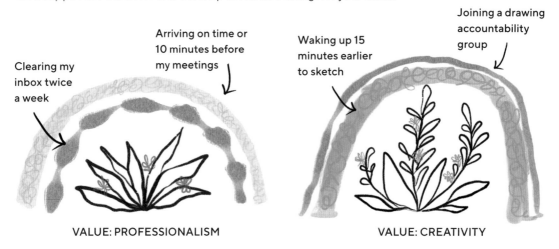

Clearing my inbox twice a week

Arriving on time or 10 minutes before my meetings

Waking up 15 minutes earlier to sketch

Joining a drawing accountability group

VALUE: PROFESSIONALISM

VALUE: CREATIVITY

Give it a try below: Choose a value to represent through the plant, and add flowers to represent your needs. Next, color in the rings above the plant to create your own arcs. Label each arc as a supportive behavior that will help to nurture your value.

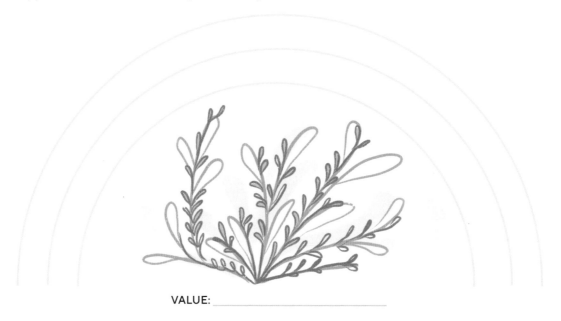

VALUE: _____

Living In and Out of Your Values

Reflect on a time in your life when you felt in alignment with your core values and a time when you were out of alignment. Explore what emotions came up for you.

Recall a time when you felt OUT of alignment with your core values. What happened?

What emotions did you feel?

What supportive actions and habits help you to feel aligned with your values?

Recall a time when you felt IN alignment with your core values. What happened?

What emotions did you feel?

What supportive actions and habits help you to feel aligned with your values?

Embody Your Values

You actively embody your values when you live them through the way you speak, act, and feel. In this exercise, you will continue exploring the art of words by lettering your values and writing them within and around your body.

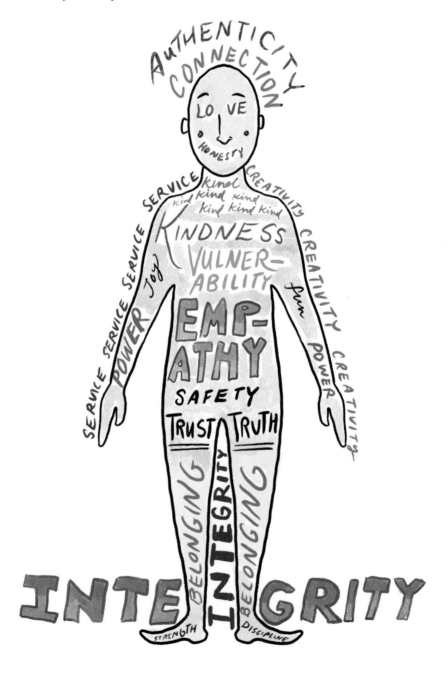

Outline the figure and fill the space inside and around it with the values you want to embody and live by. Write out the words using different colors, sizes, and lettering styles.

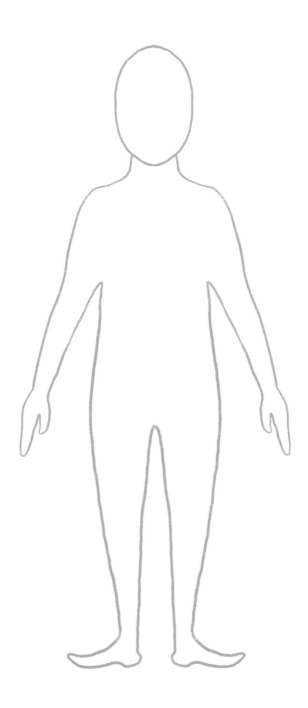

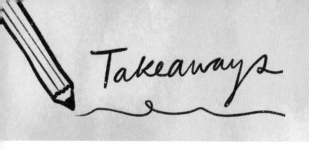
Takeaways

Reflect on your experience of chapter 8. What exercises stood out to you and why?

_____

_____

_____

_____

_____

_____

_____

_____

_____

_____

CHAPTER 8 EXERCISES

☐ Identify Your Core Values

☐ Personal Values Definition

☐ Practice Drawing Expressive Letters

☐ Express Your Values through Words

☐ Create Your Own Values Metaphor

☐ Draw Your Values Garden

☐ Behaviors to Support Your Values

☐ Embody Your Values

9

ACCEPTING
ALL YOUR EMOTIONS

change begins with
ACCEPTANCE

As we conclude our journey, you will be tempted to move into action. You will want to know how you can take all that you learned and change your feelings, behaviors, and thought patterns. But change without acceptance is empty and won't last.

In order to change, you first must accept your feelings and yourself as they are. Once you accept this moment, you can change the next.

Acceptance doesn't mean you agree with or approve of the situation. But it does mean you no longer avoid, become numb to, distract yourself from, or run away from the uncomfortable emotions you may feel. You practice accepting the moment by FEELING your feelings.

You can change, because you have sat with the reality of your emotions without first trying to change them. In this journey of acceptance, we learn the wisdom of what ALL our emotions can teach us.

American psychologist Carl Rogers says, *"The curious paradox is that when I accept myself just as I am, then I can change."*

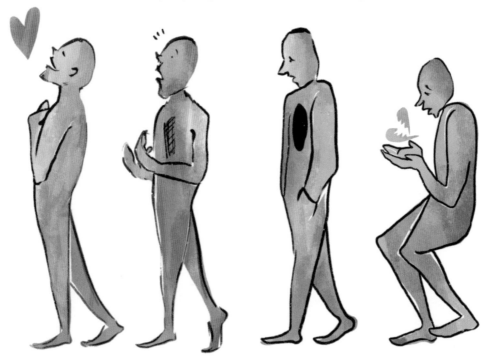

GROWING INTO MYSELF FEELS LIKE...

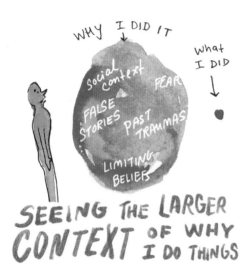

SEEING THE LARGER CONTEXT OF WHY I DO THINGS

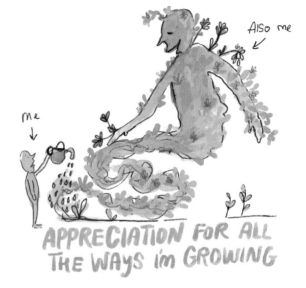

APPRECIATION FOR ALL THE WAYS I'm GROWING

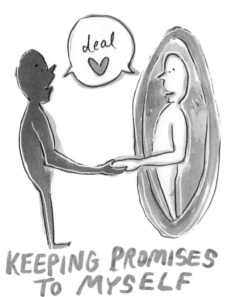

KEEPING PROMISES TO MYSELF

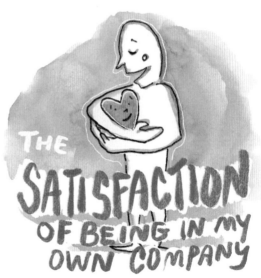

THE SATISFACTION OF BEING IN MY OWN COMPANY

In order to become the person you want to be, you first need to accept who you currently are. Even more important is to know that you are ALREADY the person you want to be. You may just be separated by layers of false beliefs, negative stories, habits, and a ton of resistance. The process of acceptance allows you to see your truest self and remove the layers of who you are *not*.

Where Do You Take Action?

If you want to practice acceptance, you have to first acknowledge *what* you are trying to accept. This comes by taking inventory of your reality: What is and isn't in your control?

The diagram below helps you to categorize four areas of your life. When you can determine when to take action and when to let go, you will gain the wisdom of acceptance.

	I TAKE ACTION	I DON'T TAKE ACTION
I CAN CONTROL	**MASTERY** Taking action on what you can control	**GIVING UP** Not taking action on what you can control
I CAN'T CONTROL	**CEASELESSLY STRIVING** Taking action on what you cannot control	**LETTING GO** Not taking action on what you cannot control

EXAMPLES:

Mastery: Exercising regularly, delivering my projects ahead of time at work

Giving Up: Finishing my novel, waking up at 6 a.m., improving my Spanish

Ceaselessly Striving: Trying to be friends with people who don't prioritize me

Letting Go: Fear of being forgotten when I'm not invited to parties

Consider which of your actions fall into the four categories below. This exercise is an initial brainstorm that you will continue to unpack and visualize in the exercises to come.

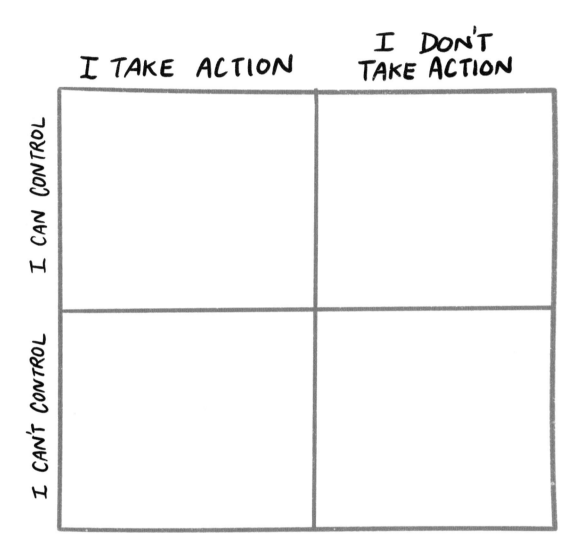

I TAKE ACTION   I DON'T TAKE ACTION

I CAN CONTROL

I CAN'T CONTROL

PRACTICE NOTICING: What feelings come up for you in each category? How does it feel to write your areas of mastery? Or of giving up, ceaselessly striving, or letting go?

177

Let Go of Your Balloons

When you gain clarity on what you can and cannot change in your life, it makes it easier to let go. Your fears and insecurities lose their power over you when you give a shape and name to what you want to release.

Fill in a few of the balloons on this page with what you want to let go of.

Types of balloons: *Below are a few examples of differently shaped balloons. Practice drawing your own in the blank space.*

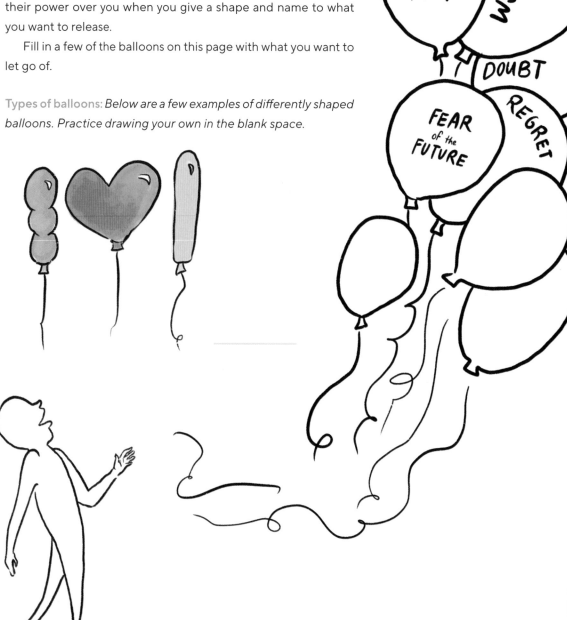

Give yourself permission to release what is holding you back. It can be harmful habits, self-doubt, false stories, toxic relationships, experiences that need to be forgiven, and much more.

Draw balloons of different shapes, colors, and sizes that float above the figure below. In each balloon, write what you are letting go of.

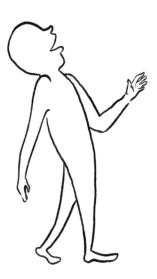

Your Circles of Influence

Now that you have recognized what is out of your control, you can shift gears and notice the many things that you *do* have control and influence over.

You have more power than you may realize. You can influence your thoughts and emotions. You can be mindful in your communication and how you show up in relationships. You can create routines, goals, and daily habits. By knowing where to put your efforts, you can even influence your future through how you choose to act in the present.

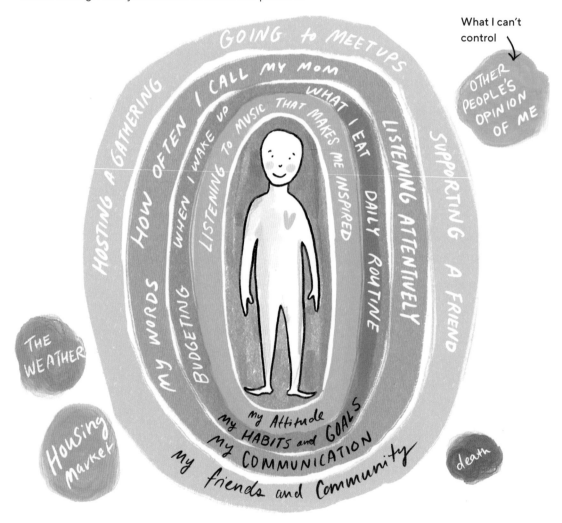

The circles around the figure represent what you have influence over.
Anything written outside of the circle represents what is outside of your influence.

Draw your circles of influence by first coloring circles around the figure. Then, with a pen or marker, write what you *can control* within each colored circle.

Start with your most personal levels of influence (thoughts and attitudes) in the innermost circles and expand from there (how you show up for others, your habits, actions, etc.).

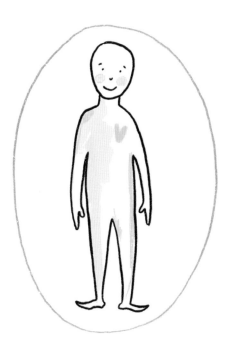

Sitting with Your Feelings

We practice accepting our emotions by feeling them. Refer to your action diagram on page 177 and recall a time when you either didn't take action when you could have (gave up) or tried to take action when it was out of your control (ceaselessly striving).

What was the situation?

Example: I never applied for the job I wanted because I didn't think I was good enough.

Example: I tried everything I could to make our relationship work, but in the end we still broke up.

What emotions did you feel?

Example: I felt regret, frustration, and sadness.

Acceptance expands your capacity to sit with your feelings without avoiding or running from them. You can also practice being present with your feelings by drawing them out as in the examples below.

Observe how the different emotions are expressed. Practice drawing your own in the blank space.

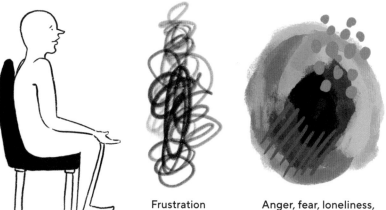

Frustration

Anger, fear, loneliness, grief, disappointment

Insecurity and guilt

"I'm not running away. I see you. I feel you. Your feelings matter. I accept you and will sit with you as long as you need. We can do this."

One way of sitting with your emotions is visualizing them on paper. Use the skills you learned in previous chapters to draw out your emotions. *Do they have a specific shape, color, line, or pattern? Can you draw them out as a body form, or as a metaphor?* Be as abstract or concrete as you like.

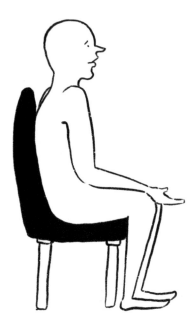

TAKE IT TO YOUR SKETCHBOOK: If you could speak to your feelings, what would you say? How do you think they would respond? Draw out the conversation in speech bubbles.

Five Stages toward Acceptance

Everyone has a unique journey toward acceptance. Letting go of what's not in your control and feeling all the emotions that come with it isn't easy. Accepting reality doesn't mean you agree with it—it simply means you will no longer avoid or run from it.

Recall a specific life situation that was challenging for you but also taught you acceptance. What happened?

Example: death of a loved one, illness, moving to a new city, going through a divorce or breakup, career change, getting pregnant, not getting pregnant, losing a friend, going bald, etc.

_____

What was it about this particular situation that you had to learn to accept?

Example: When losing my uncle, I had to accept that I would never see him again and that it's OK to grieve.

_____

_____

If you were to map out your journey of acceptance in five stages, what would they be?

Example: 1. Numbness and shock; 2. Seeking distraction; 3. Confusion about life; 4. Anger; 5. Grief

1. _____

2. _____

3. _____

4. _____

5. _____

Note: *Your journey may not be so neat and linear and conclude with acceptance, and that's OK. Maybe you're still in the middle of your journey. The purpose is for you to define and validate what your journey has looked like for you, and to recognize all the emotions you've felt along the way.*

Below is an example of what an acceptance journey may look like. The different segments of the journey are labeled with words and visualized with different lines, symbols, shapes, and colors.

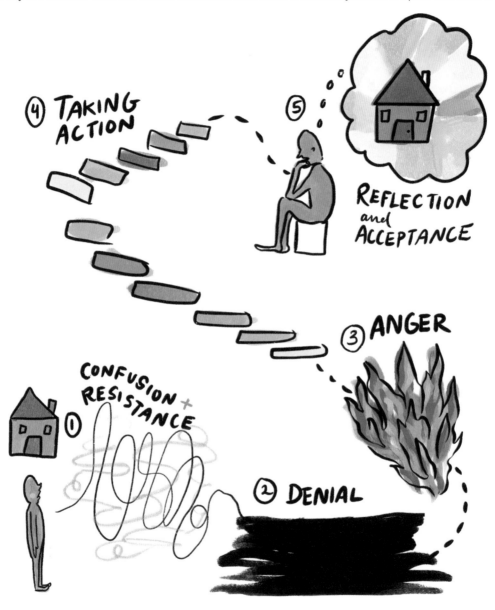

Above: My journey to accept the loss of my childhood home, which I've lived in for 25 years. *What began with a lot of confusion and resistance eventually led to denial (it's not happening), then to anger (why does this have to happen?!) and to taking action (OK, let's make this happen), and eventually to reflection and acceptance (it happened; let's keep the memory of this home alive).*

Your Journey of Acceptance

Map out your own journey by illustrating your own stages of acceptance from page 184. Begin with the small figure on the bottom left and cover the entire two pages. Each stage can be drawn out using symbols, metaphors, or even abstract colors and shapes. Label each stage of your journey.

You

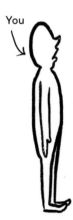

REFLECTION: Is there a particular area of your life that you are *currently* struggling to accept? If you were to map it out, where would you be in that journey? At the beginning, middle, or end?

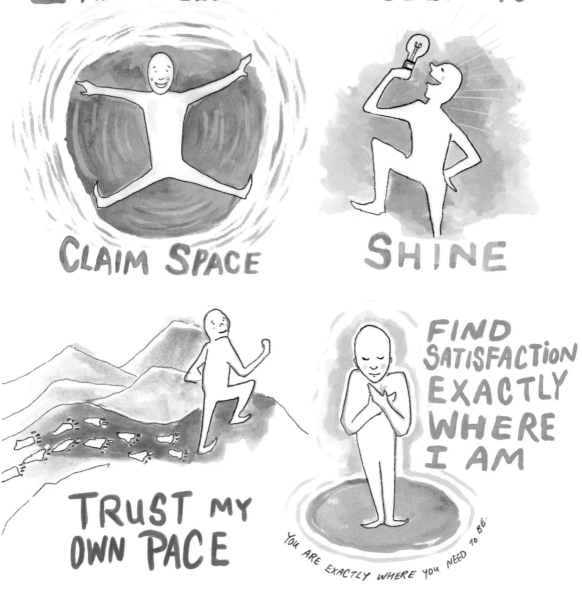

When you lean into self-acceptance, you allow yourself to shine and take up space. And most important—you can feel satisfied being exactly where you are *now*. When you give yourself permission to first BE who you are, you can then take the necessary steps to take action.

Accepting Your Strengths

Remembering and celebrating your strengths is a valuable practice for self-acceptance. Label and color the gifts on the table with your own personal strengths. They can be your warm smile, your taste in music, your ability to listen, etc. *You can also draw your own gifts of different sizes and shapes.*

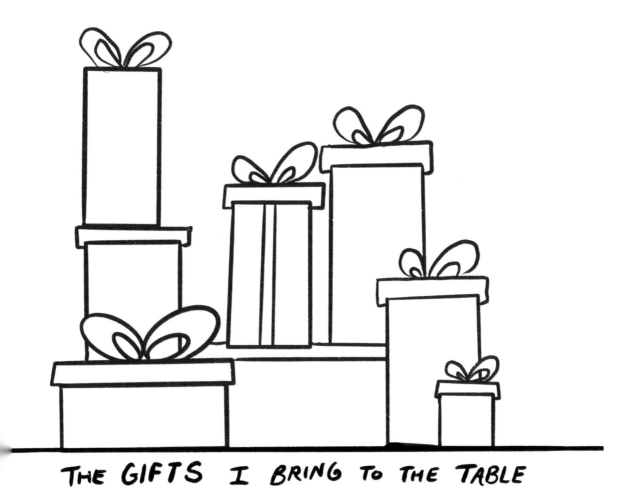

THE GIFTS I BRING TO THE TABLE

Affirming Who You Are

The culmination of acceptance is to connect back to our true *self*. To who we really are, underneath all our layers of fear, doubt, destructive habits, negative stories, etc. When we connect to our essential qualities and core values, we affirm our truest identity.

Write your own personal affirmations, or "I AM" statements, below.

Example: I am beautiful, radiant, talented, and confident. I am hardworking, determined, and focused. I am a friend, daughter, sister, and mother. I am loved, cherished, worthy, and enough. I am an artist and writer.

I am . . . _____

I am . . . _____

I am . . . _____

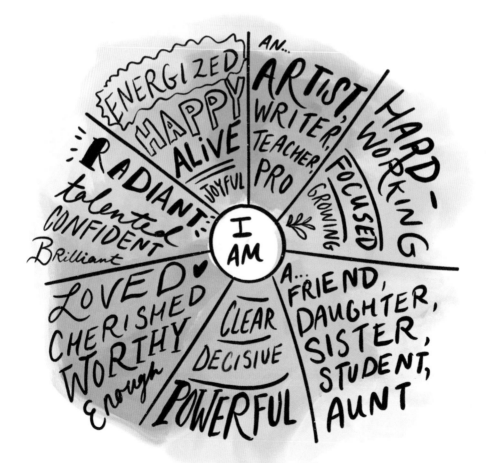

Create your own "I AM" wheel below. Color in each section of your wheel as you like, and fill it in using the values and words you want to affirm in yourself. Refer to chapter 8 for your personal values and tips on how to illustrate the words.

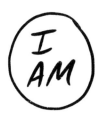

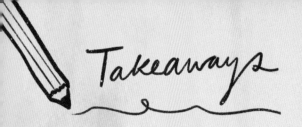

Reflect on your experience of chapter 9. What exercises stood out to you and why?

_____

_____

_____

_____

_____

_____

_____

_____

CHAPTER 9 EXERCISES

☐ Where Do You Take Action?

☐ Let Go of Your Balloons

☐ Your Circles of Influence

☐ Sitting with Your Feelings

☐ Your Journey of Acceptance

☐ Accepting Your Strengths

☐ Affirming Who You Are

10

exhale

exhale

It's easy to go through your life holding your breath. Pushing, waiting. Or you take a long inhale, consuming, learning. But when is it time to exhale?

To exhale is to find balance. Exhaling calms your nervous system and signals that you're OK.

To exhale is to rest and release. It's an active form of healing yourself and letting go of stress.

To exhale is to create space for all that you've learned and allow it to naturally settle. To integrate it into who you are. It doesn't require us to DO, but rather to BE.

On this journey of drawing your feelings, you are encouraged to take a break and exhale. To process your experience, admire your creations, and congratulate yourself before you "take your next inhale" and move on to new ventures.

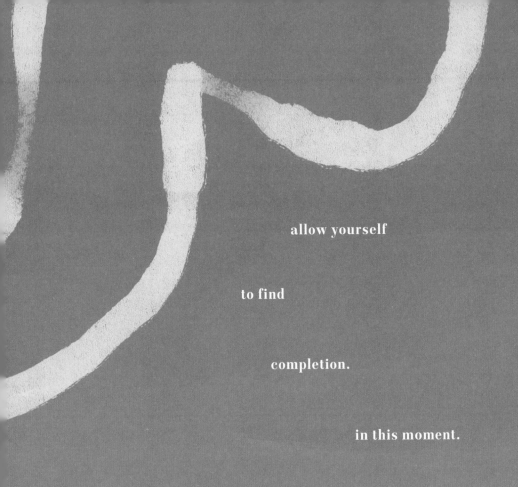

allow yourself

to find

completion.

in this moment.

in this breath.

in this chapter of life.

Mindful check-in: *What are certain expectations of yourself that you hold on to? How can you honor them and let them go?*

Affirmations for Release

Fill in the blank spaces to create your own affirmations. Practice the following breathing exercise: With every inhale, bring your awareness within; with every exhale, mentally repeat your affirmation.

I exhale and my body feels _____

_____

I exhale and my heart feels _____

_____

I exhale and I notice _____

_____

I exhale and I believe _____

_____

I exhale and I allow myself to _____

_____

I exhale and I let go of _____

_____

I exhale and I trust _____

_____

I exhale and I feel _____

_____

Three Deep Exhalations to Let Go

A guided meditation

With each of the following conscious breaths, inhale fully and let your lungs fill with air. Exhale very slowly, so you can feel the sensation of releasing your breath and letting go.

1 With the first set of three breaths, exhale fully and imagine yourself letting go of your thoughts. You can imagine balloons flying away, or clouds parting from the sky.

2 With the second breath, as you exhale, imagine yourself letting go of all physical tension within the body. You may notice areas of tightness in the body softening, almost like ice dissolves into water.

3 With the third breath, as you exhale, imagine letting go of all the burdens of your heart. These may be any difficult relationships, emotions, or anything else that feels heavy in your heart.

4 As you complete your three breaths, come back to your natural breathing and notice how you feel. Your body may feel more relaxed, your mind may be quieter and your heart lighter. Continue this exploration of conscious exhalation as long as you like.

Brach, Tara. "Guided meditation: Letting go – 9 magic breaths (5:50 min.)." October 2019. https://www.tarabrach.com/meditation-9-magic-breaths/.

The Emotions of Your Breath

Your breath is intimately connected to your emotions. Each breath carries its own feelings, stories, and memories. Take a moment to notice your breath. Is it shallow or deep, slow or fast, smooth or rough, regular or irregular? Do you tend to push it or hold it?

Recall a memory or emotional experience and note what quality of breath you had.

Example: Being in an elevator with someone I don't know   *Hold my breath and stay still*

Example: Listening to music by my favorite artist   *Breath feels light and bouncy*

_____   _____

_____   _____

The images below represent different types of emotions and the quality of breath they carry. In the blank spaces, draw the different types of breath for each emotion.

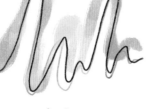

Anxious
Breathing is sporadic

Angry
Breathing is heavy and loud

Excited
Breathing is quick

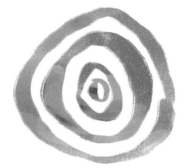

Tense
Breathing is tight and shallow

Depressed
Breathing is slow

Peaceful
Breathing is calm and relaxed

Think of a specific memory when you felt anxious and one when you felt calm. Without overthinking too much, intuitively draw and color what your "anxious breath" and "calm breath" look like.

ANXIOUS BREATH

Calm BREATH

PRACTICE NOTICING: How does the quality of your breath change throughout the day? How can you use this observation to bring greater awareness to your emotions?

Exhale as a Form of Rest

Every exhale is an invitation to rest.

Rest can look like napping. Or dancing. It can look like reading a book or watching a movie. It can look like staying in or going out with friends. Externally, rest can look like nearly anything.

Why? Rest isn't about our behavior. It's about the intention. No behavior is inherently right or wrong. It's the degree and intentionality behind it. When we lack intention, we are numbing ourselves.

When we take a behavior to an extreme, it's no longer restful. When a 25-minute nap becomes three hours long, chances are you'll feel even more tired.

When done in moderation and with the intention to relax, even scrolling on a phone is restful. But without that intention, it easily becomes numbing.

List out the different ways you numb yourself on the left, and the ways you can find genuine rest in the right column.

NUMBING MYSELF

Example: When I'm tired after work, I reach into the fridge and grab the closest sugary snack.

RESTING

Example: When I want to take a break, I treat myself by baking muffins or cookies.

resting
can
look like . . .

Allowing others
to support you

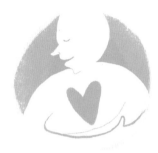

Being kinder
to yourself

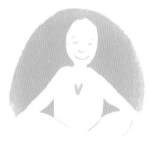

Prioritizing "being"
over "doing"

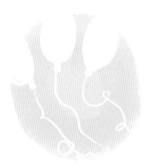

Letting go of your
expectations

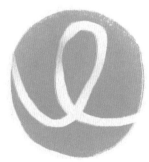

Taking a deep,
relaxing exhale

Knowing when
you are done

REFLECTION: What are some moments in your daily life that are truly restful for you?

Celebrate Your Growth

When you exhale, you make space to process everything you've learned. This includes creating space to celebrate how far you have come and all you have accomplished. Reflect on the skills, lessons, and realizations you have gathered on this journey of drawing your feelings.

What has your journey of drawing your feelings looked like? Draw a map that connects the figure to their heart. Include the lessons, skills, and realizations that you have gathered along the way.

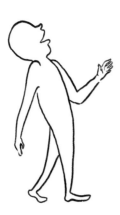

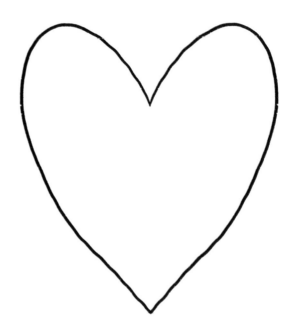

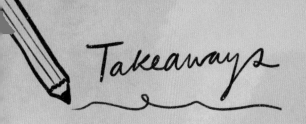

Takeaways

Reflect on your experience of chapter 10. What exercises stood out to you and why?

_____

_____

_____

_____

_____

_____

_____

_____

_____

CHAPTER 10 EXERCISES

☐ Affirmations for Release   ☐ Exhale as a Form of Rest

☐ The Emotions of Your Breath   ☐ Celebrate Your Growth

ACKNOWLEDGMENTS

 To my editor, Lauren Appleton, who took a risk on me—thank you for believing in me and this book and helping to bring it out into the world. To Anna Cooperberg for her editorial guidance and friendship.

 To Mama and Baba for always seeing the best in me and believing in me even when I don't. I'm so glad you didn't make me become a doctor, lawyer, or engineer.

 To my brothers, Nitai Ram, Balaram, and Ram Govinda, for always loving and accepting the weirdo that I am. To li'l bond, aka Kavi Krishna! I can't wait for you to read this book. To Rasa Sindhu—you are my heart's choice. Life has been a great adventure since you came.

Nithya Rajasekaran—for being my project manager, accountability buddy, and cheerleader when I needed it most.

Annie Yi—for testing out my exercises and sharing your thoughtful and profound insight.

Radha Gaasbeek, MEd, EdS—for being my therapeutic consultant when I needed it. Without you, the chapters PAUSE and EXHALE wouldn't exist.

Bhakti lata Caruso—this book wouldn't be what it is without you. You tested out every single exercise, gave your most sensitive and honest feedback, and helped me see my book from the eyes of a teacher. I'm so grateful for your help to reenvision this book.

Annameika Hopps—for helping me get started, helping me battle the inner demons of self-doubt and procrastination, and coaching me through the beginnings of my book.

 To Pranada Comtois, who reignited my enthusiasm to finish my manuscript and saw a potential in me that I couldn't see myself. Thank you for your loving encouragement.

 To Betsy and Chuck Cordes for their support in helping me through the legal contracts.

 To every single one of my students who has taken my workshops and courses. Your participation is what breathed life into this book and made an idea turn into reality!

 To my teacher, Sacinandana Swami, who inspires me to live a life of spiritual substance, depth, and devotion to God (Bhakti).

 To Srila Prabhupada and my community of devotees in Alachua, New York, and all over the world. I am who I am today because your love has nurtured me into life.

FURTHER READING

The following reading list inspired me over the course of writing this book. If you are interested in learning more about the many exercises and concepts introduced in this book, I highly encourage you to check out these sources.

Brach, Tara. *Radical Acceptance: Awakening the Love That Heals Fear and Shame.* New York: Random House, *2003.*

Brown, Brené. *Dare to Lead: Brave Work. Tough Conversations. Whole Hearts.* New York: Random House, 2018.

Kleon, Austin, and Lynda Berry. "Intentionally Spiraling Out," *Austin Kleon* (blog). February 24, 2022. https://austinkleon.com/2022/02/24/intentionally-spiraling-out/.

Lakoff, George, and Mark Johnson. *Metaphors We Live By.* Chicago: University of Chicago Press, 1980.

Lupi, Giorgia, and Stefanie Posavec. *Observe, Collect, Draw!: A Visual Journal.* New York: Princeton Architectural Press, 2019.

Schwartz, Richard C. *No Bad Parts: Healing Trauma and Restoring Wholeness with the Internal Family Systems Model.* Louisville, CO: Sounds True, 2021.

Tawwab, Nedra Glover. *Set Boundaries, Find Peace: A Guide to Reclaiming Yourself.* New York: TarcherPerigee, 2021.

Wolf, David B. *Relationships That Work: The Power of Conscious Living.* New York: Mandala Publishing, 2008.

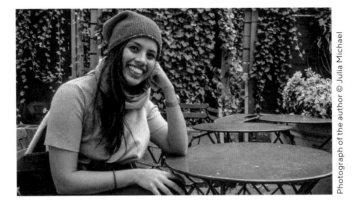

Rukmini Poddar is an artist, designer, and educator. Her creative passion lies at the intersection of emotional wellness and creative storytelling.

She began her illustration career after completing her first #The100DayProject in 2015, and has since completed this project each year for the past seven years.

Rukmini hosts regular Draw Your Feelings art workshops for large and small groups, including universities and corporate teams. When she's not busy drawing her feelings, you can find her playing peekaboo with her nephew or lounging by the pool.

She draws regularly and posts on her Instagram: @RockinRuksi